'The psychoanalysts who speak in this book, most of them, knew Laplanche personally and worked with him. They have become recognized authors around the world. The sum of their contributions gives an idea of the tremendous potential for renewal of psychoanalytic thought enabled by the reference to the General Theory of Seduction developed by Laplanche in his tireless discussion with the work and thought of Freud.'

Christophe Dejours, *M.D., full member of the French Psychoanalytic Association, president of the Scientific Council of the Jean Laplanche Foundation-Institut de France*

'This timely and necessary volume is an essential contribution to contemporary psychoanalytic thought. Through a series of compelling interviews with leading international scholars, it explores and expands Laplanche's groundbreaking ideas on seduction, translation, and the unconscious. The contributors highlight the clinical, theoretical, and ethical significance of his work, while also situating it within today's cultural and global context. Accessible yet profound, the volume invites clinicians, students, and researchers to rediscover Laplanche's insights and to pursue new directions in psychoanalytic thought. A rich and necessary resource, it keeps his legacy alive for contemporary practice.'

Virginia Ungar, *M.D., Past IPA President*

'In this polyphonic volume, Bryan Batista-Thomas gathers leading psychoanalysts from across the globe to probe and expand Jean Laplanche's audacious reimagining of Freud. Alive with energy and insight, the collection reminds us that the work of tracing Laplanche's legacy is not merely unfinished but gathering force—continuing to provoke and inspire.'

Patricia Gherovici, *Ph.D., psychoanalyst and author of* Transgender Psychoanalysis

'In this lively and immensely edifying book, Bryan Batista-Thomas has asked a diverse and sophisticated group of nine prominent psychoanalyst scholars to think about what constitutes a Laplanchean *style* of psychoanalysis. As the interviewees grapple with the clinical and theoretical implications of Laplanche's work, the reader is privy to their own styles of de-translation, translation, closure, and compromise formation. In turn, the serious reader of Laplanche is provoked to think in their own style, keeping these questions open, as they should be.'

Elaine P. Zickler, *Ph.D., L.C.S.W., Psychoanalytic Center of Philadelphia*

Readings of Jean Laplanche in Process

This book is a series of interviews with nine Laplanche scholars who expand our understanding of his work and highlight its contemporary importance and applications in psychoanalytic theory and practice.

Much of Jean Laplanche's work remains untranslated into English, but his ideas are increasingly influential in the Anglophone psychoanalytic world, especially in the United States. His groundbreaking work on gender and sexuality leads the way in terms of psychoanalytic understanding of the current social and cultural developments in these areas. This work shows the ways in which his concepts migrate and transform into a global perspective through the lenses of epistemology, clinical practice, theory, culture, and linguistics. With contributions from current members of the Scientific Council of the Laplanche Foundation and prominent Laplanche scholars, this book aims to stand alongside Laplanche's theoretical work as an example of the complexity of the relationship between theory and clinical practice.

Enriched with clinical vignettes of child and adult analysands, this book gives psychoanalysts and psychotherapists an excellent introduction to the key tenets of Laplanche's work and its application to classic and current clinical issues.

Bryan Batista-Thomas spearheaded the premier, now annual, Laplanche in the Clinic event in the United States, modeled after the *Journées internationales Jean Laplanche*. He is coediting the translation of *The Language of Jean Laplanche* (Routledge) into English. Batista-Thomas works full-time in private practice providing psychoanalysis, psychoanalytic psychotherapy, supervision, and teaching.

Readings of Jean Laplanche in Process

Conversations Amplifying Differences

Bryan Batista-Thomas

Routledge
Taylor & Francis Group
LONDON AND NEW YORK

Designed cover image: Adam Bohannon

First published 2026
by Routledge
4 Park Square, Milton Park, Abingdon, Oxon OX14 4RN

and by Routledge
605 Third Avenue, New York, NY 10158

Routledge is an imprint of the Taylor & Francis Group, an informa business

British Library Cataloguing-in-Publication Data
A catalogue record for this book is available from the British Library

ISBN: 9781032670256 (hbk)
ISBN: 9781032670232 (pbk)
ISBN: 9781032670287 (ebk)

DOI: 10.4324/9781032670287

Typeset in Optima
by codeMantra

For Justice.

Contents

Acknowledgments

I am grateful to Hélène Tessier for her steadfast support, and to the other members of the *Conseil scientifique de la Fondation Jean Laplanche/Nouveaux Fondements pour la psychanalyse*—José Carlos Calich, Christophe Dejours, Roxanne Dejours, Lorenza Escardó Zaldo, Isabelle Gernet, Udo Hock, Jonathan House, Alberto Luchetti, and Francis Martens—for their time, generosity, and willingness to participate in this project.

My thanks also to Dominique Scarfone for his participation, as well as for his supervision, mentorship, and sustained support over the years. I am equally appreciative of Luiz Carlos Tarelho and Maria Teresa de Melo Carvalho, whose patience, knowledge, and engagement enriched the work; I learned a great deal from our collaboration.

During my many trips to Paris, I had the good fortune to develop a close friendship with Nicolas Evzonas. I especially value our wide-ranging conversations, often over dinner, as well as the many hours of interviewing that frequently became late-night exchanges. His energy, creativity, and enthusiasm for life continue to inspire me.

For more than half a decade, I have studied Jean Laplanche's work in a group led by Avgi Saketopoulou, who first introduced me to it. I am grateful for her teaching, friendship, and sustained mentorship. I also thank the members of the study group, past and present—Romy Reading, Sam Guzzardi, Ann Pellegrini, Diane Fremont, Willa France, Susan Heimbinder, Adam Gaubinger, Michael Waldon, Sonia Orenstein, and Diana Moga—whose insights have continually expanded and challenged my thinking.

I am deeply indebted to Rachel Boué-Widawsky, whose supervision and mentorship supported every stage of the book process. Her incisive, creative guidance, particularly in navigating inevitable complications and maintaining momentum, made this project possible.

I am grateful to my supervisors, past and present, who strengthened my capacities as an analytic listener and helped me develop my own style: Graciela Abelin-Sas Rose, Christine Anzieu-Premmereur, Neus Carbonell, Velleda Ceccoli, Lillian Ferrari, Bruce Fink, Patricia Gherovici, Jenny Kaufmann, Janice Lieberman, William D. Lubart, James Ogilvie, Virginia Ungar, and Josh

Wolf-Powers. I also wish to acknowledge my seven analysts—D.K., G.H., J.H., J.D., I.T., K.G., and M.C.A.—each of whom, in different ways, offered me the opportunity to revisit and reinterpret experience, deepening my understanding of what it means to be human and leaving me with a lasting, generative sense of inquiry.

Above all, I thank my patients for the trust they place in me as they share their life stories. Their candor and resilience continue to teach me, and they remain central to the work.

I am also grateful to Clémence Sebag for her expertise and meticulous help with translations; without her careful work, an entire section of this book would have been excluded.

Finally, I appreciate my publisher at Routledge, Kate Hawes, for backing this project, and I thank Georgina Clutterbuck and Aakriti Aggarwal for their patient and responsive editorial support. My gratitude as well to Susannah Frearson, the first person to read my preliminary book proposal, for her early encouragement to submit a full proposal.

Introduction

This book is a collection of oral interviews from Laplanche scholars from around the world.

Members of *Le Conseil scientifique de la Fondation Jean Laplanche/Nouveaux Fondements pour la psychanalyse* (the Scientific Committee of the Laplanche Foundation/New Foundations for Psychoanalysis) present their reading and understanding of Jean Laplanche's work along with international Laplanche scholars, two of whom were doctoral students of Laplanche.

The Foundation aims "to contribute to the development of psychoanalysis in France and abroad, in the spirit which inspired the scientific life of the founder" (Admin *La Fondation Jean Laplanche*). Quarterly meetings are held to not only address issues relevant to the Foundation's mission but also offer scientific debates with outside presenters. They also organize biennial conferences whose presentations speak to the year's chosen theme from Laplanche's work. Such an event was held for the first time in Fall 2025 in the United States organized by Romy Reading, Alistair McKnight, Paola M. Contreras, and me on the topic of *Between the Message and Après-coup: The Psychoanalytic Method*.

In its form and content, this series of interviews is intended to speak to the plurality of languages and cultures of the reading of Jean Laplanche's work. As a result, there is a multiplicity of perspectives contained in this book, which can conflict, compete, align, contradict, and amplify one another. However, the arc across the chapters moves from clinical and didactic expositions to extensions of Laplanche's work, as the authors put Laplanche's thinking into direct contact with other theories outside psychoanalysis. Nearly all the chapters include clinical material, whether from the contributors' own cases or a discussion of the clinical vignettes (included below) provided to them.

The aim of this collection of interviews is not to create a synthesis or a new theory of Laplanche's work, but instead to highlight, amplify, and expand our understanding of Laplanche's work through a diverse and varied set of perspectives. These interviews examine the work of Laplanche through epistemological, theoretical, and clinical lenses.

DOI: 10.4324/9781032670287-1

Additionally, this juxtaposition of different viewpoints on Laplanche's work reveals how concepts migrate and are transformed from their original linguistic and cultural context. An example of a concept that has been transformed is "subjectivity" or "subject," which Laplanche does not use. Instead, he uses the language of "translation, de-translation, and re-translation." Another concept that has been transformed is the "Third Topographical Model," which appears prominently in some regions of the world and has been somewhat discarded in others. In those regions of the world where the Third Topographical Model is heavily considered, an entire branch of continued research stems from it. Finally, this book promotes an international (global) perspective on Laplanche's work.

These interviews raise the awareness of a 40-year gap between Laplanche's influence in France in the 1980s and the growing contemporary interest now in the United States, particularly from the relational tradition. As of this writing, not all of Laplanche's works have been translated into English. Despite Laplanche's new popularity in anglophone psychoanalysis, no books address the clinical dimension of his work nor the differences between his work and that of other psychoanalytic theorists.

A limited number of secondary texts in English show the varied ways of reading Laplanche's work while remaining faithful to the radicalness of his theory and its controversial nature. For example, some of his radicalness includes not taking into consideration countertransference in clinical practice; or that all affects are just another form of binding, such that the task of the analyst is to unbind affect from representation and increase excitation; or that the border of psychoanalysis for Laplanche is between the self-preservative and infantile sexuality, and that falling back on attachment theory pacifies this.

The novelty that these interviews introduce to Laplanche studies in the United States is to bring together a large sample size of different and complementary clinicians and theoreticians from around the world, allowing the reader to create their own theory and sense of Laplanche's work while remaining at fidelity with Laplanche's work. It allows for deviations in Laplanche's thinking to be highlighted and thus for those fault lines to become an area of further inquiry and exploration. These interviews also include clinical vignettes, which allows the reader to have a sense of how Laplanchean clinicians and theorists think through case material or do not think about clinical material.

Method

The methodology was to orally interview each contributor four to five times. The duration of each interview varied from one to one and a half hours. Some interviews ran for longer. Interviews were conducted virtually, recorded, and then transcribed. The transcript was shared with the contributor to see whether information should be added or removed and if there were factual errors. Every contributor received the same set of 14 problematized questions and three clinical vignettes (or moments). ("Problematized" is defined in the *Cambridge English Dictionary* as "to treat an idea, belief, word, etc., as a problem that needs to be examined or solved, in order to find out if it is as simple as people think.") Both the problematized questions and the clinical vignettes are on the pages that follow.

The contributors were instructed in an initial meeting to structure the interviews for themselves in the way they felt most comfortable and that the author/interviewer would follow their lead. In each subsequent interview, the questions asked would become more specific and tailored to the contributor. Once the four to five interviews were completed, they were condensed into a chapter that spoke to the central theses of this book. The interview transcripts in this book are presented verbatim from recorded conversations. Some were translated from Portuguese or French and edited slightly for clarity. Others were conducted in English. The resulting text reflects the person's natural spoken English, which might not always be correct syntactically, but which was left mostly intact to reflect the contributor's own voice and way of conceiving these issues. Occasionally, a sentence was edited for clarity. As mentioned previously, all the contributors' chapters form a kind of dialogue with one another. For this reason, this book should not be treated like an à la carte menu, but instead read starting at the beginning so that the valences of the readings of Laplanche's work reveal themselves.

Clinical Vignettes

The following three clinical vignettes (or moments) were posed to the interviewees to deepen the conversation about what thinking with Laplanche in the consulting room might appear like, whether there are specific technical differences in practice due to thinking with Laplanche's metapsychology, and to more generally introduce a clinical dimension into a discussion of Laplanche's work.

Museum Scene

An analysand goes on a date with her boyfriend. She is not fond of museums, and when she does attend, she prefers to go alone. She has mentioned this to her new boyfriend. The two take a trip together. Along the way, they stop at a known museum. In the parking lot, he turns to her with a smile and says, "I know you don't really like museums and would rather go alone. But I have two tickets for us." The analysand wonders to herself why her boyfriend made the decision for them to go there. She is partially irritated and feels that she cannot say no because it would be asserting a preference in the matter, which she has heretofore preferred not to do. She ends up attending the museum with her boyfriend.

Nosebleed Scene

An analysand had requested to reduce the frequency of the treatment due to financial concerns. The person had amassed considerable credit card debt and was unable to pay for sessions. The frame was mutually renegotiated. One day, the analysand came into session and said he was going on a three-week vacation and had bought an engagement ring. The analyst inquired how the analysand was able to go on vacation for three weeks and buy an engagement ring when he had said so recently that he was in considerable credit card debt and needed to change the session frequency. At that moment, the analysand spontaneously had a nosebleed. He bled all over his clothing and the analyst's couch and spent a large portion of the remaining part of the session standing up, bleeding into tissues.

"Sounds Like…"

An analysand struggling with a creative project that also involves working with others says that they (the person is queer and gender nonconforming) feel they have identified a core issue about themselves, something central to the treatment. They associate to the implications of this revelation and say how they would like to address it since it keeps getting in the way of their professional and personal life. They continue associating to difficulties with other people's input on the project. The analyst says, "Sounds like you're going to have a difficult time when distribution happens." The analysand flies into a frenzy. They associate after some time to feeling completely rejected by the comment. They felt the analyst was angry at them for coming to this revelation without them, and they focused on the phrasing of "you're" as though it was creating a separation between the analyst and themself. For the analysand, it was as though the "you're" was pushing them away and creating further feelings of isolation that accompanied the pain they were feeling.

Problematized Questions

1 What constitutes a Laplanchean *style* of psychoanalysis?
2 How does Laplanche's Translational Model of Repression represent a refusal of a psyche/body dichotomy? How does this refusal permeate through his work, like in the case of a radical failure of translation?
3 Related to the previous question, in the refusal of the internal and external, where for Laplanche the external other becomes the internal other, what are the implications for clinical practice? For example, how does the analyst understand the session and/or the analysand's material?
4 What are the ethics of a Laplanchean *style*? And how does this relate to metapsychology, clinical practice, and culture?
5 Which parts of Laplanchean theory are lost in translation into a different culture and language?
6 Related to the previous question, do you think that the translation of Laplanche's work into English changed Laplanche at all? If so, in what ways?

7 How do Laplanche's General Theory of Seduction and the Translational Model of Repression offer a different perspective on the clinical vignettes? Considering this difference, how would you compare Laplanche to classical and contemporary Freudian theory, Kleinian theory, Bionian theory, self-psychology, intersubjectivity, etc.?
8 In what ways does reading Laplanche in your cultural context change his theory?
9 How does the reality of the message, and the materiality of it, cause Laplanche's theory to be one that is nonsubjective?
10 Given that Laplanche did not study newborns, and his theory is not one of developmental psychology, how does his theory necessitate and work with historical foundations? Please consider both the clinical context of the analysand and within culture.
11 In what way does stressing the sadomasochistic dimension of the unconscious allow for a movement away from normative family structures and gender issues in sexuality, reproduction, and love in the common sense?
12 How do the issues of gender, power, race, and class come up in your particular cultural context as it relates to Laplanche's theory? In what ways does Laplanche's theory address these issues?
13 For you, what is an effective and Laplanchean *style* of conducting research in psychoanalysis? How is this different than in the other disciplines and in psychoanalytic research in general?
14 Do you think there are holes or incongruencies in Laplanche's work?

Contributors

José Carlos Calich is a psychoanalyst and member of the Porto Alegre Psychoanalytical Society in Porto Alegre, Brazil. He is a member of *Le Conseil scientifique de la Fondation Jean Laplanche/Nouveaux Fondements pour la psychanalyse*. Calich attempts to solve dilemmas and problems in Laplanche's work using a basis in biology, with a strong focus on Laplanche's method.

Maria Teresa de Melo Carvalho is a psychoanalyst and Professor at the Federal University of Minas Gerais in Belo Horizonte, Minas Gerais, Brazil. She completed her doctorate under the supervision of Laplanche. De Melo Carvalho was present during the time the *Problématiques* were being taught at the Sorbonne. She teaches the work of Laplanche and Silvia Bleichmar at the university and in study groups. De Melo Carvalho draws many of her reflections and theories from *Life and Death in Psychoanalysis,* and yet can take into consideration the evolution of Laplanche's thought across all the *Problématiques* and his later works. She speaks mostly about masochism, epistemology, and clinical practice. De Melo Carvalho is a member of the *Jean Laplanche Brasil* group.

Lorenza Escardó Zaldo is a psychoanalyst who completed her doctorate in Madrid, Spain, under the supervision of a researcher heavily influenced by Laplanche's work. Her entry into psychoanalysis was through the work of

Laplanche. She is a member of *Le Conseil scientifique de la Fondation Jean Laplanche/Nouveaux Fondements pour la psychanalyse*. She works primarily from a Laplanchean perspective, mostly focusing on and taking into consideration Laplanche's later work. Her discussion of clinical material is deeply embodied.

Nicolas Evzonas is a Greek Cypriot Paris-based clinical psychologist and psychoanalyst in private practice. He is a candidate to the French Psychoanalytical Association and Associate Professor of Clinical Psychology in the Department of Psychoanalytic Studies, which was founded by Jean Laplanche in 1970 at Paris Diderot University. He is the author of the book *Devenirs trans de l'analyste* (The Trans Becomings of the Analyst) and guest editor of various special issues of *The Psychoanalytic Review*, *Psychoanalytic Inquiry*, and *Studies in Gender and Sexuality*. His work on trans and countertransference is largely inspired by Jean Laplanche's theorizations on gender and put into dialogue with feminist and gender studies, where he also complexifies the notion of *après-coup*.

Isabelle Gernet is a psychoanalytic psychotherapist in Paris, France, and Professor at Paris Cité University. She collaborates closely with Christophe Dejours in her research, focusing on the psychodynamics of work, an extension of Laplanche's theory. She is a member of *Le Conseil scientifique de la Fondation Jean Laplanche/Nouveaux Fondements pour la psychanalyse*. Her work addresses non-neurotic psychopathological psychic organizations, looking at psychotic modes of functioning, narcissistic pathologies, and somatic illness. Like Christophe Dejours, she focuses heavily on the psychotic *enclave* of Laplanche's theory.

Udo Hock is a psychoanalyst in Berlin, Germany. He is a former student of Laplanche and is a member of *Le Conseil scientifique de la Fondation Jean Laplanche/Nouveaux Fondements pour la psychanalyse*. He sees Laplanche as a commenter whose theory must remain open to the outside, which is to say it should not be a Ptolemaic enclosure. Hock has the Laplanchean method deeply ingrained in his method of working. He starts from Freud, then moves to Laplanche and back.

Avgi Saketopoulou is a psychoanalyst in New York City, USA. She is a member of the NYU Postdoctoral Program in Psychotherapy and Psychoanalysis. Her work focuses on enigma, *après-coup,* and putting Laplanche in contact with other writers. She reads Laplanche from a queer, trans, queer of color critique perspective and works as an extender of Laplanche's theory. Saketopoulou expands the notion of the mytho-symbolic and its link to temporality and discusses the ways in which this affects gender, race, and class. She also discusses psychoanalytic writing and teaching in a Laplanchean *style,* and the difference between Laplanchean ethics and other forms of psychoanalytic ethics.

Dominique Scarfone is a psychoanalyst, member emeritus of the Canadian Psychoanalytic Society and Institute in Montréal, Canada. He is an Honorary Professor in the Department of Psychology, University of Montréal, where he was a Full Professor for 25 years. He had an ongoing intellectual relationship with Laplanche and was an important interlocutor for Laplanche. Scarfone sees himself as an imitator of Laplanche through the usage of Laplanche's method. He learned to be a better reader of Freud through his study of Laplanche's work.

Luiz Carlos Tarelho is a psychoanalyst in São Paulo, Brazil. He mostly takes into consideration Laplanche's so-called Third Topographical Model and expands this to consider psychosis and borderline cases. Tarelho completed his dissertation in Paris under the supervision of Jacques André. However, he maintained close contact with Laplanche during his doctoral studies. He is a member of the *Jean Laplanche Brasil* group.

Hélène Tessier is a psychoanalyst, a member of the Canadian Psychoanalytic Society, and a lawyer. She is a Full Professor in the School of Conflict Studies, Faculty of Human Sciences and Philosophy at Saint Paul University (Ottawa), Canada. Tessier is Vice President of *Le Conseil scientifique de la Fondation Jean Laplanche/Nouveaux Fondements pour la psychanalyse* and author of publications on Laplanche's work and its epistemological and ethical implications. Tessier comes from the postulate of Laplanche and focuses on the systemic nature of his theory that has an epistemology. She also stresses the sadomasochistic dimension of his work.

Postscript

In addition to meeting with the contributors mentioned in this book, I also met with Jonathan House (the US member of *Le Conseil scientifique de la Fondation Jean Laplanche/Nouveaux Fondements pour la psychanalyse*, and the editor-in-chief of the Unconscious in Translation Press, which has published most of Laplanche's work in English) multiple times. We had fruitful conversations regarding translation and his relationship with Laplanche and Laplanche's wife, Nadine. We also discussed the concept of *après-coup*, which House is quite fond of; he felt Laplanche's redefinition of *après-coup* was a valuable contribution to psychoanalysis and clinical work.

Bibliography

Admin. "La Fondation Jean Laplanche." *La Fondation*, https://www.laplanche.org/la-fondation. Accessed 2 Apr. 2024.

Cambridge English Dictionary. Definition of "problematize," https://www.dictionary.cambridge.org/us/dictionary/english/problematize. Accessed 2 Apr. 2024.

1 Lorenza Escardó Zaldo

Madrid, Spain

Bryan Batista-Thomas: What constitutes a Laplanchean *style* of psychoanalysis?

Lorenza Escardó Zaldo: When I read the question, I thought how funny, "a Laplanchean *style*." What comes to my mind first was how Laplanche loved to debate.

BBT: Debate?

LEZ: Debate. He was always in a debate. I saw him working in the *Journées internationales Jean Laplanche*, which happens biennially. It's an event where people who know his work think and discuss together in a dialogue and debate format. I think you can see it also when you turn the pages of his books that he's always in debate with Freud, with Lacan. There is an essay about Klein. But at the same time, another thing comes to my mind, and I don't know where I read it, or who told me that Laplanche was not enthusiastic about the idea of creating a school as, for example, Lacan.

BBT: It's funny in the sense of *style*, or does it feel like he would object to there being a Laplanchean…?

LEZ: Yes. I think he would have an objection with this if people started saying, "I'm Laplanchean."

BBT: While he says that and I read that or someone has told me something similar, that he was not an imperialist—he didn't want to make a school. However, his theory is very rigorous, and it's well problematized and systematic. How does one sit with a dialectic of not wanting to be imperialistic, not wanting to be a school, but having a theory that is difficult to integrate with other theories, that almost demands a certain purity to it?

DOI: 10.4324/9781032670287-2

LEZ: I think there is a Laplanchean *style* of psychoanalysis but that Laplanche actively refused to constitute a school, which was more related with Lacan. I think that was because of Laplanche's proximity to Lacan—being his protégé in a way. Or maybe he had a humble sense of self. He always preferred to say that his work was founded in Freud. Therefore, he said he's a *"faithfully unfaithful"* Freudian.

However, I do not think that the General Theory of Seduction is a difficult theory to put in contact with other theories. We have seen fruitful contacts with attachment theories (Dornes, 2002) or with gender theories (Saketopoulou & Pellegrini, 2023), for example. On the contrary, Laplanche and his psychoanalytic procedure par excellence, I mean the *step-by-step procedure,* have left within our reach throughout his texts each step of its elaboration, problematization, and systematization. It bequeaths a theory to its possible refutation but also to debate and confrontation with other theories.

BBT: Clinically, do you think that there's a Laplanchean *style*, a particular way of working?

LEZ: Yes. I believe that clinically there are several hallmarks of a Laplanchean *style*. Because Laplanche says that, for him, the analytical situation is the most important part of Freud's discovery.

Laplanche's theory develops or points out an "original seduction" that he later called the Fundamental Anthropological Situation. He locates the transformative potential of psychoanalysis in the reactivation of the "original adult-infant situation" within which the analytic situation operates.

We want to *reactualizar*; we seek *reactualización*.

BBT: Reopening. *Reactualizar* would translate to "reopening of."

LEZ: A reopening of the original and thus universal adult-infant situation. I think a Laplanchean psychoanalyst has this always in mind. When you start a process, you are trying to make this reopening possible.

You are always keeping in mind that in the best of cases, you will rebuild this original situation for your patient and for this reason that you'll always keep thinking of the differences between the psychoanalytical situation and the original situation (Escardó & Golergant, 2012). Let us say that what is reactualized or better yet reopened, in the analyst-analysand situation, would be the inevitable adult-infant asymmetry. The analyst is the adult (introducing asymmetry); the patient is the child (the *hermeneut*, the translator). For Laplanche, this asymmetry is essential, even foundational.

Regardless of this analogy, I think that the psychoanalytical situation and the original situation imply some important differences. First, we have the psychoanalytic method, which essentially is a step-by-step procedure, which the adult who takes care of a child doesn't have in hand. Therefore, I think a Laplanchean *style* in clinical work is one that feels safe because the analyst knows that he can rely on this method. On this basis and in light of this model, one is well equipped to better understand.

It is a style based on the idea of reintroducing the essential asymmetry that characterizes the original situation, but also on the idea of containment—both in balance to move toward an encounter with the traumatic.

BBT: You are describing the situation in the consulting room as there being a safety, which Laplanche discusses in *New Foundations for Psychoanalysis* in the "Practical Task." There, Laplanche discusses having a sort of consistency, being benevolent, and how these qualities allow for *le baquet* [the tub]. You just said it allows a reopening of the traumatic. Could you say a little bit more about what you mean by that?

LEZ: When you create this safe space with the frame, with regularity, you are at the same time allowing for more of the strange, *lo más ajeno* [the off thing] to come through the consultancy. I think the traumatic is to get in contact with your unconscious, and, further, the unbound and the untranslatable.

BBT: The attack of the *Sexual*. Encountering the *sexual* death drive.

LEZ: Yes, and the *sexual* death drive is the result of the impact on the individual, and subsequently on him or herself, of the encounter with another, an adult who does have a sexual unconscious, as discovered by psychoanalysis.

It's not easy to talk about this Laplanchean *style* in clinical work because it's an important mixture between being there for your patient, but at the same time to be neutral, holding the silence, "*se refuser*" from adaptive needs. To not always be responsive is central in our clinical perspective, as it is central to the patient as far as possible to hold the fundamental rule, free association.

I am aware that this aspect of the analytical function is strongly rejected nowadays, and here, in Madrid or in other working and supervisory groups, when you try to explain this point of view, the centrality of asymmetry, it's very commonly associated with the figure of a cold (classic) psychoanalyst. You start to say that it's not at all the case. However, more importantly than to be neutral is the renunciation—the analyst's refusal to take up a position of knowing, while still being the adult other to whom meaning is attributed in the repetition of the Fundamental Anthropological Situation. There is also explaining how important it is to allow the hollowed-out transference. Going further, balance is important, and to let things happen so that the unconscious, alterity appears. In this way, we will be able to solve, analyze, and dissolve the enigmatic messages.

BBT: What would it look like when alterity, the unconscious appears?

LEZ: For me, it's when the patients get in contact with something that is difficult for them. Some aspect that the person doesn't know about or is not known and scary to them.

BBT: Could you say a little bit about your experience as someone starting out mostly having a background in Laplanche's work and then reading other authors and then coming back to Laplanche? Seeing the otherness of other authors through the lens of someone who has a background in Laplanche, instead of the reverse?

LEZ: I started reading Laplanche in a seminar group. Then when I started reading Laplanche, for me it was quick. I needed to read other authors that taught me about Laplanche. Because, only Laplanche was a little bit like "Wow." I needed to get far from him through knowing other authors. I started to learn about Dominique Scarfone, Christophe Dejours, Jacques André, some Brazilians who were working closely with Laplanche doing their doctoral work in Paris. For years I was reading Laplanche and these other authors. They were working with the theory of Laplanche from different points of view, in their own interest. These authors helped me to read Laplanche. It was after these years reading when people said to me maybe it could be interesting if I read André Green, or if I read other contemporaries of Laplanche. I started to do it, and it was interesting. But I cannot tell you now about the conclusion of this work. I feel it was really enriching to get far away from Laplanche and then go back to Laplanche's works. In this moment, I'm just getting back to his works. I will think a little bit more about this.

BBT: Most people start from a foundation elsewhere with Freud, Klein, Winnicott, Bion, Lacan, at least in this country, the Intersubjectivist, Relational School. What I find interesting is that what you did is effectively go the reverse, but also have contact with the other. You're having contact with another author who is another and then going back to Laplanche and seeing Laplanche through a different vantage point. I guess what's interesting about that vantage point is not just, "I see that Klein works clinically in this way or that Stephen Mitchell works clinically in that way," but also there is a particular vantage point difference when you're now in contact with the other. It's almost like I'm conceptualizing it as though you have the unconscious of the other being a different author like Stephen Mitchell attacking the Laplanche ego, something like that.

LEZ: My own Laplanche ego also. Because now when someone attacks Laplanche, you feel someone attacking your little Laplanche ego. But for me it's been always like this. I wrote my dissertation for my doctorate on the unconscious *enclave/enclaved* unconscious. A topic which interested me greatly because it provided new insights into the non-neurotic branch of pathology. There were authors that were working closely to Laplanche, pushing him to go far and to redevelop new topics. He started to reopen, to rethink a new topic, and subsequently built a new foundation. Later in his life, he started to develop dialogues with other authors, like Christophe Dejours (1986, 2001) and Luiz Carlos Tarelho (1999). After some time, the notion of intromission came. I think it was Dominique Scarfone (1994) that started to really push him in that direction. These new topics at the last years of his work! I think his life was always this dialogue with other authors. In this line of a Mitchellean unconscious attacking a Laplanchean ego, we could think of the work of dialogue and debate as a way of linking this drive attack motion.

But as you speak of Stephen Mitchell or relational psychoanalysis, I find it interesting to note that Laplanche was a French psychoanalyst who transmitted his theoretical work instead of his clinical practice. Laplanche can be more easily related to "classical" practices or focused on the purely intrapsychic. Although undoubtedly, and especially, the most unpleasant and less bearable aspect is his defense of the asymmetry in the analytic duo, as I explained earlier.

For the last three years, I have been participating in a group in Madrid with colleagues from various theoretical orientations. We have been working with different authors of Anglo-Saxon relational psychoanalysis, paying special attention to differences in clinical practice oriented from this relational theory, and psychoanalytic work that is more classical. I find it very interesting because we are always moving in margins, in the borders. In some ways, we tackle the question, how to sustain/welcome asymmetry so that otherness becomes present without abandoning presence or containment?

BBT: I wanted to take us back to something. Can you make a finer differentiation and highlight similarities between the analytic situation and the Fundamental Anthropological Situation? Also, how would it reveal itself clinically?

LEZ: Sure, you had asked me about the reopening and what was traumatic in the analytic situation. I'm thinking here about the encounter with our unconscious, and what exactly the experience of that is. I was thinking about what exactly the otherness is—or the traumatic encounter. It is something we find, a thing that is opposite to the subjective, our subjectivity. A functioning of our more anarchy-like aspects where the economics of the *Sexual* has no limits on its demands. It could be traumatic to discover you have this economic functioning of the *Sexual*.

BBT: Can you say a little bit more about what you mean by the economy of the *Sexual* and the no limits demand of it?

LEZ: I believe that we are already talking about an operating mode at work in all the topographical levels, corresponding to the economic dynamic of drive forces at play in the psychic conflict—the bound and unbound forces (with conversions from one form to another) in the different levels of our psyche and in which in extremes or poles we find the most detached, the most extreme, the most radical aspects of our functioning, whether in the pole of disinhibition or in the extreme of rigidity (Laplanche, 1994).

All of this is to say that this otherness is the unconscious, the arrival of the final point, when a message gets into translation. You have the aspect that achieved translation, and the aspect that does not and goes into the unconscious. This is the otherness, the *corpo externo interno* [internal foreign body], which Laplanche liked a lot. He referred to it a fair amount at the beginning of his writing. It's placed there like a splinter, the source object of the drive, of the *Sexual*—in whose domain a different regime governs, based on an economy of excess, of a "more and more," that is never exhausted, never satisfied.

You asked me a little bit about the difference between this otherness, the unconscious after the translational process, and the otherness related to the *enclaved* unconscious. As we discussed, the writings of Laplanche are mostly focused on the former.

If we turn now to the second of your clinical vignettes, the one with that spectacular symptomology of the nosebleed, we can think that it is more related with something that is not connected with the sexual unconscious. In the "Three Meanings of the Term 'Unconscious,'" in *Freud and the* Sexual (2011a), Laplanche discusses a topographical model, where there is the conscious-preconscious related with the sexual repressed unconscious, and the unconscious *enclave/enclaved* unconscious. We can think that maybe the comment touched upon something that is enclaved or more related to the *enclaved* unconscious. We can see that with this bleeding, we are facing the difficulties for psychic elaboration in your patient, his little capacity for symbolization. The bleeding, in a way, was like a reaction, a direct reaction after he received the question.

I was thinking about the renegotiation of the frame, how this change was presented to the patient, and what was it about this negotiation, given it was on the self-preservative level. Which is to say, the issue of the fee, the problems with the credit cards, and on the other side is the level of the drives. The analyst and the analysand agree to allow the self-preservative to pass, and more attention to be paid to the drives and fantasies. I was thinking to myself why allow the self-preservative to take place? I am not sure what to make of the change in the frame. Whether to understand it as resistance or something else. Given we are always trying to push the self-preservative out of the frame, how did you feel making this change in the frame?

We are always attempting to stay on the level of the drives in the frame. This is of course quite difficult. It is also important to maintain a balance as we were saying before, because if there are only the drives, it explodes. The session and treatment explode, but at the same time if we fail to sustain the valuable asymmetry, the refusal position in the analytical process is not established. Did you agree with him without taking issue? Did you speak with him about the need to reduce the frequency as a need to escape?

BBT: Initially, I just went along with it. I didn't interpret. I didn't inquire. I went on the self-preservative level. At the second time, when the patient returns saying that he was going on vacation, and he was buying an engagement ring, and then I sort of inquired but was still on the self-preservative level. I don't think it was on the level of fantasy, or the drives.

LEZ: I was thinking about the role of the analyst. What is interesting in this vignette is that it helps to look at the analytic situation in two ways. The analysand and the analyst. I was asking in part if you were working with resistances, because when he came, he said he was going on vacation, he had bought this ring, and you ask him about how it's possible. I found some aggression in this comment. That you were perhaps angry.

BBT: No, I was not angry.

LEZ: With making a long interpretation like this maybe you were pointing fingers in the highlighting of what was going on.

BBT: I said in a neutral fashion: "Can you help me understand how you are able to go on a three-week vacation and buy an engagement ring, when you told me just a month or two before that you were in a lot of credit card debt, and you needed to change the session frequency?" That's all I said. Then he bled. I wasn't angry. I was more perplexed.

LEZ: Can you imagine that he feels an aggression in this comment?

BBT: I don't know how he took it; it's possible. Are you asking in a sense how he understood the message?

LEZ: Yes.

BBT: Possibly, he could have understood it aggressively.

LEZ: When I read this question, what I felt was it was a message that was a little raw.

BBT: It's very intersubjective. You're listening to how the message is being understood by the analysand through their response. Is that how you're thinking of it?

LEZ: Yes.

BBT: Given that his response was to have a symptom, to bleed, do you think that was something of a failure of translation?

LEZ: The message, the question or inquiry you made, passed through, and arrived to impact him in such an aggressive way that he responded with this bleeding. There are no defences. This makes me think of the unconscious *enclave* and how these messages get into the psyche directly. Normally, the sexual unconscious is better protected with the preconscious or the conscious. Here, there is an intense question from the analyst and impressive response. This leads me to think that contact was made with something less protected and, with it, a contact with something that is of the content of the unconscious *enclave*. There's no distance.

BBT: I never thought of the unconscious *enclave* as not having defences in the same way as the sexual unconscious. Does Laplanche write this or is this your thinking?

LEZ: In *Freud and the* Sexual (2011b), Laplanche uses the expression *"à fleur de conscience"* to describe how the unconscious *enclave* is maintained only by a thin layer of conscious defence (p. 201). But as we said before, he develops this notion with the inestimable help of other authors, like Marta Rezende Cardoso. This Brazilian psychoanalyst wrote her dissertation (1995) about the superego around the time of the publication of *New Foundations for Psychoanalysis* (Laplanche & House, 2016, p. 135). This is when Laplanche had started thinking about those superego messages that cause little *enclaves* in every one of us. These developments are a clear precursor to the unconscious *enclave/enclaved* unconscious and this new topographical model called the *troisième topique,* the Third Topographical Model.

You can imagine the person lacks some capacities for symbolization. I would think that you are being cautious with him, being close to him, working in small pieces. Because he can have a decompensation. I was thinking about what we would call this work. Since I think this patient is at the beginning and making an important step toward being in an analysis. At the beginning, you are working with him to build a psychic conflict. What do we call this work? If you start the analysis proper, which is to say, de-linking, you break him down and this will make him quite anxious. Now, we can say that the treatment is moving more in a psychotherapy sense than in an analytic sense.

I was also thinking about considering this bleeding as a symptom, as you say, or following this perspective, the unconscious *enclave* as not having a symptom but a beautiful example in which the ego is confronted with the unconscious *enclave/enclaved* unconscious, whose irruption into the space of the ego provokes, as its principal defense, a violent appeal to the body, either through the somatic or through the act.

BBT: Much of the time I make psychotherapeutic interventions. Occasionally, I may make an analytic one depending upon where the patient is psychically, because there is a fair amount of variability. Sometimes he can be quite out of reality, and at those points I cannot make an analytic interpretation or an analytic comment. It would just make the situation worse.

LEZ: But you feel like you're able to work in these two levels. You are feeling that you are working also in neurotic levels?

BBT: Sometimes and sometimes no.

LEZ: I fear I may be jumping too far or maybe putting my desire of seeing more in your analysand or in this clinical vignette of yours than is really happening.

BBT: You are bound to fill in, to fantasize, to interpret in some way the vignette and my analysand. The interest is what is the relationship between theory and practice in a Laplanchean sense.

LEZ: OK, now turning to the third vignette. The point where I start my reading of this vignette is the transferential reaction of your analysand. I perceive an intense transferential reaction that leads me to feel that this is the kind of patient with whom you must work a lot in the transference. You will have an experience completely different of what transference is, and opposite from other patients. In my experience, you have some patients where you struggle, or you have the feeling of a labile and intense transference; and with other patients, it settles in, but in a more secure and stable way.

I think it's an interesting vignette; it marks for me the optimism that can be made in psychoanalysis or psychoanalytic psychotherapy. "A new translation of the unconscious enclaved always remains conceivable" (Laplanche, 2011b, p. 310). That is a quote from Laplanche. The more optimistic Laplanche.

In my view, we can see that you're working—this is a little bit abstract but, you're moving in two different levels of otherness. On the one hand, the classic internal foreign body, the repressed sexual unconscious. And on the other, a more radical otherness that is even more external and alien to the patient.

For it seems in the vignette, in the more classical Laplanchean sense, the work of the de-translation has been satisfactory. You are helping him to make some de-translations, so he can make new, more open translations. I say that because in that moment the analysand appears very happy with identifying this core issue, like a new representation, something central for the treatment. For me, the analysis has constructed something that will help the treatment move in a more authentic way. A significant gain for your patient's professional and personal life.

This work could represent a more classical way; parts from the sexual repressed unconscious now came up to enrich the consciousness or the self. There is movement happening in this person, to his ego, to feel more, I don't know, powerful in a way. To start thinking it's possible to live their personal and professional life with more authenticity. It's my interpretation.

But this also implies a movement in the other side, in the *enclaved* unconscious. If we continue following Laplanche, we must think that when we help someone to de-translate or de-link, which is our job in the most psychoanalytic sense, to open the analysand to make de-translations so that he can later make richer and more flexible new ones. While the psychotherapeutic position, as I was saying earlier, is more based on establishing or stabilizing existing translations. Ideally, we move to de-translation, make de-translations, but that also implies that pieces or parts of this broken translation will go back or return to the *enclaved* unconscious, where they will remain until a new translation is possible, for new material to be represented.

BBT: Can you say a little bit more? What do you mean, "it goes back to the *enclaved* unconscious"?

LEZ: Normally, how I understand it, when you de-translate, you are breaking apart meaning. What could no longer be in the conscious part of the mind goes back to this space, the unconscious *enclave*—waiting for new translations.

We also have messages in the unconscious *enclave* that are quite violent. For this reason, many authors say they prefer not to call them enigmatic messages but, instead, something on the order of psychotic, perverse or paradoxical messages. These messages will produce a radical failure of translation. In my point of view, I don't know if I really like the terminology, but these paradoxal or brutal messages that will maybe never attend a translation are nevertheless waiting, blinking in the *enclave*.

We also have enigmatic messages that are not as brutal as the previous type of messages but compromised by the sexual unconscious of the adult. Nevertheless, the infant receives it in a moment that could not be translated and thus generates *enclaves or an enclaved* unconscious. They will wait in the unconscious *enclave/enclaved* unconscious until translation is possible. Earlier on in his work, when the distinction between implantation and intromission was not already established, Laplanche called it the *psychophysiological skin*. A stock of untranslated messages, temporarily awaiting translation. A translation that can only be initiated by *reactualización,* or reopening.

Therefore, we have three possible ways, and we are talking here about the possibility that, in the time you are helping your patient to de-translate, this temporarily enriches the unconscious *enclave*. Because of the continuity that this model proposes, a message previously translated and had, in this extended process, undergone the path of the ego and the sexual unconscious.

As you help your patient to break this translation (always two-sided; with the side that implies more stability to the ego or preconscious, and the side that implies the continuity of sexual repression), that de-translated message then cannot remain in this zone and becomes part of the *enclaved* unconscious.

For me, that's a strong moment in our therapies or analyses. There is a fair amount of excitement of the unconscious *enclave* because it must be noted that the major de-translating action of the cure temporarily enriches the stock of messages to be re-translated and re-symbolized. This can allow for movements in the treatment, but at the same time, depending on the level the patient is operating at, it could lead to a breakdown or decompensation.

It is a difficult step to follow. You point toward a work to de-translation, de-linking. But if what is in the air is de-linking or, to be clearer, if the death drive predominates, we do not know what can happen. This makes me think again of your patient and this strong transferential reaction and what there may be in it of the action of an unlinked drive. I feel it a little bit like that, maybe you don't, but I feel like this fly of rage makes you wonder what is being touched, what has come into play, and what kind of message the patient is dealing with? In many ways, you are in a privileged moment.

BBT: Why do you say that?

LEZ: Because by launching this movement of de-translation-translation, perhaps some of the unconscious *enclave* will be able to move into the more neurotic area of functioning, into the conscious-preconscious/*Sexual*[1] sector in this Laplanchean unified model.

Dominique Scarfone, among others, has continued to develop this path opened by Laplanche and has worked on the idea of a traumatic "blow" in the context of the cure to establish a true *"après-coup"* that, once elaborated, establishes a real past and mitigates the current pain of the trauma.

BBT: You drew a differentiation in the topographical model, between the classical sort of unconscious with the preconscious, repressed unconscious, and the *enclaved* unconscious, which is larger. Mentioning also how they work in parallel. There's an image of this in *Freud and the* Sexual. You were saying that the two of them exist on a continuity between one and the other, and as a clinician you need to take into consideration both. Clinically, what would that look like to consider the both of them working, and to work with the two in parallel, or think clinically with the two of them in parallel? What would you listen to? What would you consider?

LEZ: For example, I'll discuss a patient of mine and a moment when I feel this is occurring in the analytical situation. When constructing the topography, the movement will construct an ego and an unconscious

> with conflicts and defenses. I feel like the patient in some way is structured in this conflictive or neurotic way, which was functioning well, with a good capacity to associate and to bring dreams and thoughts. There were some issues around identity, but we were always working with this possibility of restructuring in a conflictive topography. In some parts of the treatment, she came for some sessions, and she lost this capacity for thought, for association. Sometimes she could not even talk and sometimes she came with strong expressions of affect—anger. But she was not capable of thinking about this anymore in a conflictive way; she lost the capacity to work on a more neurotic level.

It's like being with someone who sometimes can show you how she is being constructed. I imagined her in these moments like an infant, a child, receiving all these messages from the adults around her. She can do this work of translation with something going into the ego; it is part of her consciousness, and other parts that she loses will remain in the unconscious.

Everything is going on, and she starts functioning on a neurotic level with very little difference. But in the other way, when she comes to session with this incapacity of talking about or hearing this in a conflictive or neurotic way, I start thinking about all the structures that come from this other kind of message that could not establish the process of translation and psychic differentiation. They will remain in the unconscious *enclave,* but they probably never are translated. But I have also wondered at certain times, in certain treatments, what relationship these jumps or decompensations might have to do with the activity of the analysis itself. I am referring again to how the de-translation will momentarily increase the stock of material to be translated and how the patients can withstand that pressure or that load.

Returning to the case of this patient, I have asked myself if it's something about the treatment and all this work of de-translation that we do that causes her to have these moments. Sometimes it is a lot for her to have to deal with; it's like the sleeping "something" of the unconscious *enclave/enclaved* unconscious or the increase in stock of messages to be translated might be somehow overwhelming to the ego. It's when, I presume, she becomes without capacity, in an extreme passivity, like being an infant.

I think we are always structuring, restructuring in the relationship with others. Everything starts from the Fundamental Anthropological Situation. I'm always thinking in regards to my patients that when they are being confronted with the enigmatic message, it will be the normal General Theory of Seduction. But I'm always concerned also about in which forms they're being confronted by the traumatic seduction. What I like a lot about Laplanche's work is when he thought about traumatic seduction, it's not restricted to sexual abuse but to the overwhelming impact of adult sexuality in the child. Danish psychoanalyst Judy Gammelgaard (2014) has highlighted the usefulness of this position in her work with her patients.

BBT: Can I just clarify? You're not talking about intromission; you're talking about implantation still?

LEZ: No, when I started talking about the traumatic seduction, I started speaking of intromission.

BBT: Okay.

LEZ: Yes. But, in intromission there are also degrees.

BBT: Can you say a little bit more about the degrees of intromission?

LEZ: It's about this debate I mentioned in the beginning. At which moment do we stop talking about the enigmatic message and directly start calling it a perverse message? When you talk about implantation, you are talking about messages that are compromised with the sexual unconscious. When we are talking about intromission, we are not anymore in this degree—because we are not anymore with a message that is compromised, which is part of the repressed *Sexual* but, rather, something that is more on the level of the unconscious *enclave* of the adult. It appears suddenly in a brutal form.

BBT: Laplanche says that the message is just violent.

LEZ: It is violent. There is something that didn't have this work of translation. But the difference is maybe that the two of them could be part of the unconscious *enclave*.

BBT: I just wanted to go back to what you were saying in terms of the patient that you were referring to—the idea that you do the work of de-translation and then suddenly there are moments when the patient cannot speak or, you didn't use the term, becomes a little psychotic. But there's something different, strange. Something a little strange goes on, and your hypothesis is that it's the *enclaved* unconscious and that you need to be careful because it could lead to what I understood as a breakdown. You didn't quite say that, but it's simultaneously a precious moment because something is going to come out of it, but at the same time it's a risky moment because the patient could have a breakdown.

I think of how we started out by saying there's a continuum of something that's more neurotic to something that's not neurotic. I think it could be very easy from the outside to pathologize this and say that the patient is borderline, for example. I don't know if this patient is borderline or not, but it would be very easy to pathologize the symptomatology and the structuring of the patient as being borderline, as compared to saying that this is a normal function of the treatment. In the de-translation something is coming out that's altogether new and unknown to the both of you—the analyst and to them, the analysand. That might be curing in the treatment and it's the otherness, it's something that's completely alien, different to the patient, but that's present nonetheless. This is an interesting movement and articulation.

LEZ: Yes. Balance. I was speaking about balance. For me, the more years I work, the more I really appreciate this precious and risky moment. When you are working in a position where you are more focused on reinforcing already-existing translations, elaborations that the patient gave himself at a given moment, it is maybe safer, less pressured, less risk.

BBT: It's just reinforcing the ego.

LEZ: Yes, just reinforcing the ego. There is less place to allow the otherness.

BBT: I think this is something that would be nice to return to because I think it's very different than what is conceptualized as psychoanalysis. Psychoanalysis, I think, is a little bit more supportive in some ways like Relational Psychoanalysis or other forms of psychoanalysis as compared to what Laplanche is talking about, or even what you are referencing, which is something that is both risky and precious—of getting into these states of what sound like very big dysregulation.

LEZ: Dysregulation.

BBT: When the drives are so present in the consulting room.

LEZ: Maybe it's just a more intimate and personal view, the way I experience it. In any case at such moments, it is useful to remind oneself as well that the infant, the human, is a natural hermeneut. I think again how balance is an important thing; and Laplanche always points this out when he says that in every psychoanalytical process, there must be psychotherapy moments.

Note

1 Referring to Laplanche's later conceptualization of the sexual unconscious.

Bibliography

Dejours, C. (2001). *Le corps d'abord*. PUF (Original work published 1986).

Dornes, M. (2002). *Psychanalyse et psychologie du premier âge*. PUF.

Escardó, L., & Golergant, D. (2012). Situation anthropologique fondamentale et situation analytique. Réflexion sur leurs différences. *Journées Internationales Jean Laplanche.*

Gammelgaard, J. (2014). Seduction and the problem of translation in the context of sexual abuse. In *Journées Internationales Jean Laplanche: Cerisy, 2012.*

Laplanche, J. (1994). Les forces en jeu dans le conflit psychique. In *Journées Internationales Jean Laplanche: Canterbury, 1994.*

Laplanche, J. (2011a). Three meanings of the term unconscious. Edited by John Fletcher. In *Freud and the sexual: Essays, 2000–2006* (pp. 246–271). The Unconscious in Translation.
Laplanche, J. (2011b). *Freud and the sexual*. The Unconscious in Translation.
Laplanche, J., & House, J. (2016). *New foundations for psychoanalysis*. The Unconscious in Translation.
Laplanche, J., & Mehlman, J. (2015). *Between seduction and inspiration: Man*. The Unconscious in Translation.
Rezende Cardoso, M. (1995). *Surmoi et théorie de la séduction généralisée*. Université Paris 7 – Denis Diderot.
Saketopoulou, A., & Pellegrini, A. (2023). *Gender without identity*. The Unconscious in Translation.
Scarfone, D. (1994). Ma mère, ce n'est pas elle: De la séduction à la négation. In *Colloque international de psychanalyse: Montréal, 3–5 juillet 1992* (pp. 97–106). PUF.
Tarelho, L. C. (1999). *Paranoïa et théorie de la séduction généralisée*. PUF.

2 Udo Hock

Berlin, Germany

Bryan Batista-Thomas: As Laplanche's former student [from 1991 to 2012], what changes have you seen in his intellectual tradition and thinking? What are the impacts of these changes on his metapsychology and thus clinical practice?

Udo Hock: I can start with my reflections. In my view, you can differentiate three periods in the work of Laplanche. The first period is when he is still a kind of pupil of Lacan. We know for certain that he was in analysis with Lacan for a very long time, from 1947 until 1964. The first period starts with his earliest texts and ends with the termination of his analysis in 1964.

I would say in this period, Lacan was the decisive person insofar as Laplanche wanted to find answers to questions which came from Lacan. You have his text with Serge Leclaire, *The Unconscious: A Psychoanalytic Study*, where Lacan's question is in the middle: Is the unconscious structured like a language? Another text from this period, a book, is *Hölderlin and the Question of the Father*, where Laplanche works around the question: Does the formulation of Lacan's *la forclusion du nom du père* [the foreclosure of the name of the father] work for understanding what goes on in the life and work of Hölderlin? Can it explain the psychosis of Hölderlin? In the third text, *Primal Fantasy, Fantasies of Origins, Origins of Fantasy*, co-authored with Jean-Bertrand Pontalis, Laplanche, in my view, attempts to find an answer to the question of the relationship between structuralism and psychoanalysis.

BBT: You were saying Laplanche was asking questions in relation to Lacan. Questions where Lacan had left off. Do you think it was Laplanche's way of making a differentiation from Lacan?

UH: Yes.

DOI: 10.4324/9781032670287-3

BBT: Do you think it's in some ways a response to the analysis or do you think it's an intellectual differentiation?

UH: I can't know if it's a reaction to the analysis. But he introduces new turns. He didn't follow when Lacan said, "The unconscious is structured as a language." He turned the phrase of Lacan around and said, "The unconscious is like—a language, but not structured" (1979) as well as "The unconscious is the condition of language" (1959). But when you change a formulation, you remain bound to the formulation in a certain way. You can see, when you read this text, that Laplanche didn't follow Lacan as others did it in that period. You can see that Laplanche, together with Leclaire, search for their own way to Freud.

Laplanche was preparing to leave Lacan in this text, *Primal Fantasy, Fantasies of Origins, Origins of Fantasy*. Lacan was the one who raised the questions, but Laplanche didn't appreciate the solution he had found in writing on Original Fantasies for a very long time. Later in his work, he changed his mind on the Original Fantasies. He thought there were no inborn fantasies in the human mind. Everything that is within the unconscious comes from the other. There is no mythological, no biological, no phylogenetical unconscious in mankind. This discussion, inspired by Lacan, about a possible structure of the unconscious is, for me, the first period of Laplanche.

The second period begins for me with the *Vocabulaire de la psychanalyse* [The Language of Psychoanalysis]. It includes also *Life and Death in Psychoanalysis* and *Problématiques I–V*. What is characteristic for this period? I think, first, he has abandoned Lacan. He took the opportunity to organize a new group, the Association Psychanalytique de France (APF), together with others. He abandoned Lacan and tried to find his own way back to Freud. The formulation is not *retour à Freud mais retour sur Freud, sur l'oeuvre de Freud.* i.e., *I've got to return, not return to Freud, but return to the work of Freud* in a certain way. Less the person. Laplanche didn't like it when people had arguments in which the concept of transference had great value. He didn't like to say, "I was in transference with Freud." He didn't speak in that way. Lacan did. Laplanche was interested in the work; the person did not matter much to him. Together with Pontalis, he wrote *The Language of Psycho-analysis,* and he found the first axis; perhaps he didn't find it in that book, but afterward, in *Life and Death in Psychoanalysis,* he found in a certain way the axes or let's call them axioms, which were interesting to him. In *The Language of Psycho-analysis,* he couldn't choose. He was the person who brought all the pieces of Freud together in that work. But afterward, in *Life and Death in Psychoanalysis,* he found the major axis, which oriented his work toward Freud.

BBT: The axis being the self-preservative and infantile sexuality?

UH: The axis is first sexuality in all its manifestations. I would say, in *Life and Death in Psychoanalysis* (1976), you can find the first book on the primacy of sexuality in the unconscious. I would say, in that book, the primacy of the other had not been established. But you can find formulations in Laplanche at the beginning which tend in that direction. The primacy of sexuality, this is in *Life and Death in Psychoanalysis*. Then comes the series called *Problématiques*. What is interesting here is that he works on Freud's notions of anxiety/Angst, castration and symbolization, sublimation, the unconscious, and transference. He analyzes Freud with Freud in a certain way. However, I think that in this period, he doesn't invent many new ideas. I would say all these first *Problématiques* turn on the language of Freud. He doesn't insert very many of his own ideas.

BBT: Would you say that he stays close to the epistemology of Freud?

UH: No, I wouldn't say that. However, I would say, very early some premises of Freud are rejected. For example, the phylogenetical hypothesis: Laplanche doesn't affirm it from the beginning. Perhaps only in the Original Fantasies. He looks around, searches. He isn't sure how to anchor the unconscious. But in *Life and Death in Psychoanalysis* and in the *Problématiques*, you won't find passages affirming phylogenesis or biologism in the unconscious. I have never found any passage where he uses biological arguments to explain the functioning of the unconscious. Freud sometimes does, and insofar it's not the epistemology of Freud, but Laplanche looks around in Freud with a specific method.

BBT: In *the Unfinished Copernican Revolution*, Laplanche has the essay "Interpreting (with) Freud," and you used a version of that saying, "analyzing Freud with Freud." Are you saying that he's using Freud within himself, Freud with Freud, in exploring specific concepts. Is that it?

UH: Yes, that's right. He looks, for example, for a notion like *l'angoisse* [anxiety]. He hasn't a fixed theory at the beginning. He looks through the texts of Freud and he tries to find the passages where Freud isn't very clear. He likes to find passages where Freud isn't clear. Freud says in that text this, and in another text, he says that, and that's not the same. There are, let's say, not oppositions, but confusions; there are open questions. That's what I mean in saying "interpreting Freud with Freud." You are not very fixed on the solution but on the questions. It's not most important to find an answer to an open question. It's much more important to formulate the question and see where the question takes you. The *Problématiques I* is a very thick book, 300 pages or more. Laplanche takes each sentence of Freud seriously, each passage, each article.

BBT: I'm thinking of a couple of things that come later in Laplanche's work. Where, for example, in "Goals of the Psychoanalytic Process," in

Between Seduction and Inspiration: Man, he says it's for you to have a question, but the purpose of analysis is not to cure the patient, it's just for the analyst to not have a goal in mind. It sounds almost like a clinical position I'm hearing in this method of working with the texts, working through the *Problématiques*. I'm also thinking of the *Problématiques* almost as being a technique. If one could say it that way.

UH: Yes, I think it's very good idea to compare it with the clinical situation. You do not choose very quickly what you understand. But you hear it, you follow the patient, you follow the text without choosing too fast how you understand it. That's how I understand Laplanche. Perhaps we need more information from the patient. We need more information from Freud and his theory on anxiety or castration. That's how he works in this second period.

Perhaps you can say it's the same technique as in Freud's *Interpretation of Dreams*. The same technique, epistemology of the clinical situation. This is the second period. Eventually, Laplanche chooses. He is not interested in everything. He chooses some notions, and he tries to redefine them in a certain way. Question of anxiety, castration, and so on. The third period is the period with his so-called Seduction Theory. Is it the "Generalized Seduction Theory" in English?

BBT: "General Theory of Seduction."

UH: There he says that's my new foundation. It's really the French word, *nouveaux fondements*, it's the same in English, new foundations, in German *neue Grundlagen*. That's really a big word, the basis for psychoanalysis, and for sure he formulates his own theory. It's not Freud's theory anymore. It's Laplanche's theory. He begins with many new ideas, I would say. For example, *transference en creux* [hollowed-out transference], etc. He began earlier with these notions, but now they spread all over his work. He makes less commentary on Freud, and until his death he works on his own theory. Some people say that he often repeats his core theory. During this last period, he looks for new solutions to problems which are quite ancient in psychoanalysis, like sublimation, masochism, and so on. In *New Foundations for Psychoanalysis*, he presents his theory in a completely systemized way. It is very pedagogic. It's a kind of pamphlet. This third and last period lasts from the middle of the 1980s until 2007. He ends his publications in 2007. He didn't write in his last years.

BBT: There are people who tend to stick more with one time period versus another. I know within the Scientific Committee, some members think that the *Problématiques* era was better than his later era and so on. In what ways do you see how working with theories and Laplanche's thinking from a specific era would affect clinical practice, or his understanding of metapsychology?

UH: This is a complicated question.

BBT: Yes. Just one caveat: I know it can be understood that I'm asking about the person. But I'm not asking so much about the person. But how the understanding of let's say *Life and Death in Psychoanalysis* as the pinnacle of Laplanche's thinking, without taking into consideration that he later changed his mind, affects the understanding of his work. For example, if someone sticks with the notion of étayage [leaning-on] without moving onto the General Theory of Seduction.

UH: In a certain way, in the last period, you can see, more clearly than in his earlier periods, if this or that is or isn't contradicting the theory. Laplanche is quite clear in saying the unconscious comes from the other, and that it is sexual. All these ideas are quite univocal, becoming more of a system. Although he didn't really like rigorous systematization. For him, thinking should be an organization open to change from within. However, eventually he did systematize and enclose his own thinking. In the earlier periods, it was never so easy to say what he was thinking or, saying something a little differently and remaining open to ambiguity.

BBT: I've heard multiple times that Laplanche was not an imperialist. He did not want to create a tradition, a school, a framework, the way that Lacan did. Yet you are saying his later theories are systematized. How can we understand this dialectic?

UH: For me, Laplanche in a certain way has always given comment on Freud. What are the consequences for everyday work? For example, in our *Vocabulaire de Laplanche*, we give notions to everybody, and everybody must write about the notion. I have written about "leaning-on" and "source-object" for example. For me, it's always connected to Freud when I write about Laplanche. For me, it's not a theory on its own. There are others on the Scientific Committee who, when they write about a notion, do not make references to Freud. They stay within the work of Laplanche. I prefer to take Freud and to say afterwards, "What did Laplanche say about Freud and the solutions you find in Freud?" This is for me the difference within the group. Others say it's not so important—we are writing about Laplanche; you can skip Freud. I say to all the people who work in that group, please begin with Freud, and then explain what Laplanche is doing with Freud. This is a concrete example of how I work with Laplanche.

BBT: It's interesting, because you are maintaining almost a dialectic between Laplanche and Freud and moving back and forth between them. That way it doesn't become Laplanche as an enclosure. It's almost as though you are creating another for Laplanche, as though it were Freud. They are constantly in dialogue.

UH: Yes. Let's do things in such a way that notions become or remain fluid. That they don't fix something, but that they stay in movement. You can say I like to insert Freud in Laplanche and vice versa. But for me, Laplanche and his work are not a theory on its own, in a certain way.

BBT: No, it's interesting in many ways because what you are making me think of is the exigency, the source-object.

UH: Yes.

BBT: You mentioned Laplanche as a theorist is not meant to be alone.

UH: I said that you're right.

BBT: How would you conceptualize that?

UH: For me, it's a theory which is based on the work of Freud. In a certain way, I'm not very happy when people enclose Laplanche in his own theory. They say, "Here Laplanche says this" and "Here Laplanche says that, and this is not the same," and so on. I'm not so sure why they work in that way. I'm not so interested in knowing all these differences. Because, for me, it's more interesting what he is saying about Freud. You know, when you stay in Laplanche's own work, you cut the work from the body. For me, Freud is the body. What Laplanche says about Freud is more interesting than drawing a circle around his own theory. He does not stand on his own in my view.

BBT: He writes somewhere that his work is an experiment, an experience. His texts are an experience, and, in some ways, I hear that in the conceptualization, the experience of the importance of the body that you make.

UH: I knew Laplanche for a very long time. Longer than Hélène Tessier [knew him]. Much longer than Jonathan House, and so on. Christophe Dejours had known him for a very long time because they were in the same psychoanalytical association. I truly appreciate Laplanche, but not as someone who has created his own theory. It's a commentary on Freud, which has become a "new" theory.

BBT: It's interesting since, in some ways, it can't be its own theory because if it becomes its own theory, it seals itself up and it's not open to the other, which is counterintuitive to what his theory is about. I'm now going to pivot: Do you have any thoughts about *Après-coup: Problématiques VI*, or any thoughts about the concept of *après-coup* in general in Laplanche's work and method of thinking?

UH: The first point, a very important point, is the question of translation. For Laplanche, the question of *après-coup* and the question of translation were linked together; you can't separate them. He says it at the beginning, and he says it at the end of the *Problématiques*. For him, the

German word *Nachträglichkeit* is a kind of example for the translating process, which you can compare with the translating processes in the psyche.

You have a word, and you don't have a good translation at the beginning. "Something" is more than your capacity to find a good word. You can compare it with the task of a child who hears something that he can't understand very well. He must find ways of comprehension—ways of translating what he's hearing but doesn't understand. That's one of the examples that comes from Freud, the example of the Wolf Man and perhaps also Emma. Linguistically, the German word *Nachträglichkeit* is very interesting, because Freud created the noun, *Nachträglichkeit*—this word didn't exist before Freud. But *nachträglich* is a common word; it's like "post scriptum" or "afterwards." The English word "afterwards" is nearer to the word *nachträglich* in a common sense; and Laplanche, in his book, really tries to find a good way to make differentiations in the concept of *Nachträglichkeit*.

One possible translation is "afterwardsness" instead of "deferred action." Laplanche looked very closely at the translation of James Strachey to find out which words he used for his translation ("afterwards," "deferred action," "subsequently," and others). He took up the most important passages in which Freud spoke of *nachträglich* and *Nachträglichkeit* and looked at how they were translated by Strachey. What is so revolutionary about that pair of words? I understand it as something that happened in the past, which will be changed in the future. That's not the normal course of time; things happened in the past, and they are over. But to me, this is the most important thesis of Freud on the unconscious—things are not done in the unconscious; they come back in the future.

BBT: What do you mean "things are not done in the unconscious, they come back in the future?"

UH: I think Dominique Scarfone invented the English word, "the unpast." Things are not in the past; they are always present in a certain way.

BBT: The now, now, now.

UH: (There is only one now.) In my view, the unconscious doesn't know the past—the past and the unconscious are incompatible. Like in the dream—in the dream, you have one time—it's the present, you don't have the past in the dream. You can read Freud's *The Interpretation of Dreams* and you will find that he says that in dreams, there is only one temporality: the present. In the chronological way of thinking, *Nachträglichkeit* is a way to bind together the past and the future. The so-called past will, of course, influence the future, but the future will also influence the past. In my view, this is the normal way in analysis in each session, but you won't conceptualize it in that way, because you are not used to thinking in that way. In a certain way, by means

> of *Nachträglichkeit*, chronological time is overcome or cancelled. The so-called "timelessness of the unconscious" is put into effect. We continue to speak of "past," "present," and "future," but under the influence of the *Nachträglichkeit*, they start to waver; they are no longer separated from each other. Take the formula "return of the repressed": Where does the repressed come from? It comes from the future, you discover it during your personal psychoanalysis, it's not archived in the past, like in a library.

All the examples from *Problématiques VI* illustrate the fact that the past and the future are linked together, that they are interwoven, and in a certain way, you are in the middle of this tension between past and future. For me, the best example is one from *The Interpretation of Dreams*, which I will cite now:

> Love and hunger, I reflected, meet at a woman's breast. A young man who was a great admirer of feminine beauty was talking once—so the story went—of the good-looking wet-nurse who had suckled him when he was a baby: "I'm sorry," he remarked, "that I didn't make a better use of my opportunity." I was in the habit of quoting this anecdote to explain the factor of "deferred action" [*Nachträglichkeit*] in the mechanism of the psychoneuroses (SE 204).

That example comes from Freud and Laplanche. I like this example very much, because here you can see the tension. You see the tension between the baby and the adult, and the interdependency of both. I'll explain what I mean. You have two or three possibilities to understand this situation. The first possibility is to say, in the Jungian way, what does this man do? He takes his fantasies as an adult and projects them into the past. In the text of Freud, if you say, "If I had thought," then it's an *irrealis*, which is the grammatical expression in German. It means this is a time which hasn't existed—*if I had known*—so it's essentially an imaginary time, a time of a retrospective fantasy, which comes pretty close to the young man's own interpretation. By the way, in this context, the translation of Strachey's "deferred action" doesn't fit at all. The ladies' man just regrets that nothing happened when he was a baby at the breast of the wet nurse. In his own view, there is no "action" at the beginning; the good opportunity has passed and he did not make use of it.

Laplanche is not very happy with that interpretation, because he says, as Freud will do some years later, the baby himself has his own sexuality, infantile sexuality. What about the erotic pleasure the baby senses when sucking on the breast of the wet nurse? Isn't that the first erotic experience, which Freud describes in extenso in his *Three Essays on the Theory of Sexuality*? We are psychoanalysts; we think there is infantile sexuality, which shows itself in this moment. Let's change the first interpretation. Let's say in this situation sexuality, more exactly infantile sexuality, comes from the child, and what the young man is saying is a repression of the pleasure which existed in that time. The accent is more on the sexuality of the infant, not so much on the sexuality of the adult.

The third interpretation comes from Laplanche, who says both interpretations are wrong—the most important interpretation involves the woman. This woman is responsible for the sexualization of that situation, because Laplanche says, at the beginning, there is no infantile sexuality, infantile sexuality is not innate, and sexuality comes from the other. It's the primacy of the other, and in a certain way, this child is hystericized by this woman. This woman will libidinize the baby—without the breast of the woman, there is no infantile sexuality. There is the beginning of the meeting of the sexual other in that situation, which is always very difficult, because we are small babies, and we don't have the psychic apparatus to really be a partner for that big woman who gives you the breast. We profit from that situation, but there will be a legacy of that situation, which returns later in our sexual life as adults.

What does it mean? This sexual life as an adult is always conflictual. That means you won't find long-lasting satisfaction; you fantasize, because you are always in that conflict between an infantile sexuality—which is polymorphic and perverse—and this task as an adult to find a new object outside your infantile sexual world, which is never the right object; it's always a substitute.

You have this early experience with your mother, or with a substitute for your mother. After puberty, it's necessary to leave this incestuous world where you have met people who are your mother, father, sister, brother, and you must go out in the world, outside of the incestuous universe. Then all the objects you will meet, in a certain way, are substitutes. You're allowed to live your adult sexuality, but in a certain way, they are not the original objects you are looking for. Of course, you can't stay inside; you must go outside. The solution is not that you stay in the family, because this is psychotic. The solution to go outside the family is a kind of compromise, because the first meeting with that maternal object is, of course, forbidden—by law, by psychic inhibitions. I think that in the words *après-coup*, *Nachträglichkeit*, the conflict that you have is spread out; you see that your relationship to your own sexuality is always conflictual. You won't find a solution which will be satisfying for eternity. There is always a tension between too early and too late, which is well illustrated by the anecdote of the woman lover.

BBT: The conflict that you were describing in relation to going out to find a new object, I don't know if I've ever heard anyone discuss objects in relation to Laplanche except for part-objects, and the totalizing objects, which he was not in favor of. How would you situate Laplanche's thinking regarding objects?

UH: You can link it to my example by saying, first, you are the object before you are the subject. Look at the situation with the baby and the mother—you are, in your unconscious, the object of what your mother will do with you: how she will give you the breast, how she will feed you, etc. For me, this is the first important point—when we discussed with Laplanche twenty-five years ago the question of object relationships, he always said, "You like object relations theory, okay, but you have to say, as a baby, *you* are the first object, the object of your mother." I would say this is very close to Lacan. Then, in the second step, you try to find your own object; but first, you are an object of implantations which come from the other—the enigmatic messages.

This is my first answer—I am the object of an unconscious, of the other, which is stronger than I am, and which is full of repressed sexuality. On the other hand, I, as a baby, am born without any sexuality and subjected to the sexuality coming from the other. But you will develop, and I would say that Laplanche is talking about the part-object, but also about the total object. If I'm right, he thinks that the total object is more or less a question of how you can integrate the *sexual* death drive. I think the *sexual* death drive for him is very much linked to part-objects, and the binding force of your life drive is more linked to the *sexual* life drive.

That's my answer to your question about objects in the work of Laplanche. You are, in a certain way, at the beginning in a situation of helplessness in front of forces that come from the other, and you must do your best to translate what's coming from the other. In the story of that baby and that mother, sexuality is linked to nourishment, and you must find answers to the excitement taking place in that situation, and which perhaps stays in your body, in your mental apparatus. For example, your ability, or lack of ability, to have a good relationship with a woman/partner depends on your capacity to make good translations. When you are overwhelmed by the excitement that comes from your childhood, you can't find a good way to relate to others, like in the major psychopathologies.

BBT: With this in mind, maybe we can pivot to the vignettes. Did any of them stand out to you?

UH: Yes, I read them with great interest. For me, the nosebleed scene is the easiest vignette, although I don't know why. As you describe it, the unconscious of the patient becomes visible. We must think on it, but it's not a question of interpretation. You have a kind of reality, a breakdown in the reality, which shows that the unconscious of that patient expresses itself. In the other situations, it's not so easy, but in this vignette, for me, it's very clear. When someone asked Laplanche, "For you, what is the unconscious?" He says, "You have an accident, and you break your leg." This was an example he gave, and this nosebleed scene is quite similar in a certain way. There is a scene which is very difficult for the analysand, and he can't react in another way. Your intervention, for him, was not well translated. It's a translation which doesn't come to a better end.

BBT: A better end in the sense that it can't be translated into a better translation?

UH: Better end means that he can speak, that he can say something to you, that he has other possibilities to react. He can become angry, he can say, "What's up here?" But that would be a better translation, less suffering. It doesn't mean that he gives you an answer which is very eloquent; it means he gives you no other answer than to produce a symptom. His answer, it's a symptom for me. Translation doesn't mean that he gives you the right answer. You have no right answer, but it would be an answer which doesn't produce this very exciting reaction. It would be a better answer if he could be angry. If he said, "What do you mean? Who do you think I am? All my confidence has gone away with what you are saying. What have I done wrong?" You can give many answers. But he's shocked; that's why his nose is bleeding in my mind.

BBT: There's something Hélène Tessier said, which I'm curious as to your thoughts on. Hélène commented that I spoke outside of the tub, and that I was moving away from his fantasies and making a comment that was on the level of the self-preservative, would you agree with that?

UH: I agree.

BBT: Can you explain a little bit more?

UH: If you make a comment, you give an intervention. You can say, on a self-preservative level, "Let's talk about money." But inside this comment, you provoke many things which have to do with money, but also, "Am I a liar?" "Who am I for you?" "Do you want to destroy me?" Out of the tub means it's not an intervention which allows you to continue to be in balance—you are shocked.

Sometimes you think, *Can I say that?* Perhaps this person will feel blamed. This patient might not be capable of giving you his feelings in another way. You couldn't see, or smell, his anxiety; you didn't have a psychological feeling about his instability in that moment. That's very interesting for the process. He speaks with his nose bleeding; he doesn't speak with words. I think it's very interesting, and I like your example, because I always like when the psychic reality meets material reality, like in your case, material reality meeting external reality. The other examples are okay, we can talk about them, but here, you really have the unconscious speaking, in my view. For me, what you said is, for your patient, a kind of enigmatic message, which shows its impact by the symptom he produces. It's not enigmatic in itself, but it's enigmatic in the effect which it provokes. When you say something to your patient, you can't know if what you're saying is an enigmatic message; you only know it by the affects you provoke.

BBT: I don't know that I ever conceptualized it that way, but it makes sense because you don't know what's enigmatic because of your repressed unconscious. You can't say, "Oh, I'm sending out an enigmatic message." I don't think I ever connected the two, but I completely agree with what you're saying. You are listening to the patient's response; it's not about the analyst, that's why countertransference in a Laplanchean framework doesn't make sense. But I think in what you're saying, as it being enigmatic to the patient, I agree completely.

UH: It's the same logic as in the traumatism. You can't say what is traumatic for someone outside his own reaction to what is going on. You might give someone your hand for too long, and they think this is a sign that you've fallen in love with them, and you say, no, that's wrong. By the way, Christophe Dejours totally agrees with me that, in the end, it's the patient who is decisive regarding these questions: What is enigmatic? What is intrusive?

When you stay inside the tub, people don't normally lose their balance; it's like a dream which allows you to keep on sleeping. Of course, these sessions are very helpful; it's our everyday life as psychoanalysts. It's a special moment when you are outside of the tub. You will learn more about the unconscious of the patient. You can compare this situation to a dream from which you wake up. But we can go into detail about nose bleeding—what is nose bleeding? It's like you opened the skin. You opened the kind of protection he normally has, and you don't have good protection against bleeding from the nose. I think nose bleeding is always a kind of excitement which is too great to hold.

BBT: What would you say about transference, if anything, in that situation? The hollowed-out or the filled-in transference.

UH: It's not so easy to give an answer to your question, but perhaps it's a kind of hollowed-out transference, because you don't know exactly what happened, and he doesn't know what happened. It's not a transference, which is easy to understand. It might have something to do with your own enigma. I don't know, but you can say it's a kind of transference effect. If I said the same sentence to this person, he would say, "Well, it's interesting what you are saying," but it wouldn't have the effect it has. Perhaps you can say it has to do with a hollowed-out transference because the enigmatic aspect in that scene is quite considerable. It's not that you say, "I am this one for you." This would be a filled-in transference, and he is bleeding. But you don't know, and I don't know exactly why his reaction is so pronounced.

BBT: I'm curious as to your thoughts on leaning-on and the abandonment of leaning-on and the implications of that. Also, as a member of the Scientific Committee, where do you notice people misreading Laplanche or his reading going astray? It could be in Germany, but just sort of in general.

UH: Let's start with the question of leaning-on; it's the easiest question for me because I have worked on it for many years. The central text is *Problématiques VII: Le fourvoiement biologisant de la sexualité chez Freud*. Is it translated into English?

BBT: It's *The Temptation of Biology: Freud's Theories of Sexuality*.

UH: You can say that the whole book is on that question, the theory of leaning-on. Do you know this theory well?

BBT: More or less. It's been a while since I studied it, but if I understand it, the basic premise is that you have attachment, and from attachment, sexuality peels off.

UH: Yes, that's it. You can find the roots in Freud's *Three Essays on the Theory of Sexuality* (2016). The theory of leaning-on says you have the self-preservative instinct and the sexual drive, and in the original situation of being fed by the mother, the two drives, or instincts, coincide. The mother gives her breast to the baby—we had this example for *après-coup*. *Après-coup* and the leaning-on theory are closely linked in the theory of Laplanche. You have the self-preservative instinct and the sexual drive, and the theory of Freud means that, in giving the breast to the baby, infantile sexuality originates. This is the most important part of the theory of leaning-on, and Laplanche worked on that theory for a very long time. In *Fantasme originaire* (1965), I don't know if he first conceptualizes the theory, but he begins to analyze the notion of drives in psychoanalysis. He writes long passages on the origin of infantile sexuality, and at the end, he says, how can it be that the mother gives her breast to the baby, and by miracle, infantile sexuality is born?

After several decades, he concludes that this theory doesn't fit. The theory is wrong; it's nice, but it's a narration, it's a kind of myth, which is my word. He changes his attitude vis-à-vis the origin of infantile sexuality and says it's from the mother's sexuality that the infantile sexuality is born—that primal scene of sexuality. Without the sexuality of the mother, there is no infantile sexuality of the child. This is a strong thesis, but as each decade goes by, he is more and more persuaded that seduction theory is the truth in the theory of leaning-on, because seduction means for him that, in getting the breast of the mother, the baby is seduced by the repressed sexuality of the mother. Without a mother or another person who sends his or her sexuality to the baby, there is no infantile sexuality. My interpretation is that the theory of leaning-on is an intermediary space for him to articulate his seduction theory.

You have three possibilities for explaining the origin of infantile sexuality. Some people say that infantile sexuality is inborn, the Kleinians, for example. You have this intermediate theory of Freud, which I call the theory of leaning-on. Then, you have seduction theory, which is the solution for the incongruencies in the theory of leaning-on. Since we don't think that infantile sexuality is inborn, how can it be that in giving the breast to the baby, infantile sexuality arises? You only have one solution—you have to say it comes from the other. It's okay to call this the theory of leaning-on, but *only* when you admit that the sexuality comes from the other. You must admit that infantile sexuality is not created, but it was already present in the caregiver.

BBT: You said leaning-on is a kind of myth. I'm surprised by that. Can you explain how leaning-on is a myth, and your thoughts on how Laplanche realized that?

UH: We had a small congress last year in France and we discussed this problem, and one of my colleagues affirmed the theory of leaning-on is not a myth, so we don't all have the same opinion on that problem. But most of us think that it's a myth because this theory wants to explain the origin of something—the origin of infantile sexuality. Questions of origin are mostly explained with the help of myth. *Les fantasmes originaires* [original fantasies], leaning-on theory—all these theories try to explain the origin. *Les fantasmes originaires* try to explain many questions which have to do with origins: the origins of fantasy, the origins of sexuality, and, in a certain way, the origins of life. *Le fantasme originaire* of the coitus between parents is the myth of how we come to life. I call the leaning-on theory myth because it's a way to explain the origin of something, but in fact I don't think the explanation works. That's why I call it myth.

BBT: It sounds like it took Laplanche two decades to move away from leaning-on, and you're saying that some members of the committee think that it's a myth. You said what makes it a myth is that it's trying to give an originary point to something. My question is how do you differentiate culture and myth from scientific thought and theory in psychoanalysis?

UH: Laplanche thinks of the myth in one way. He says the myth is a narration that gives an answer to enigmatic messages. It's an answer, but you won't find a good answer—it's a kind of infantile theory, which is my translation. Like children, there are many questions that adults don't know how to resolve: how the earth began, is there life after death, and so on. Laplanche thinks that the myth is quite like theories of children who try to find answers, but not in a scientific way.

Laplanche was a very scientific man, and he said the myth is not scientific. We try to give answers with the help of metapsychology, and it tries to analyze the function of the myth, but it's not mythic itself. Metapsychology is not a mythical thinking. He creates the notion of the mytho-symbolic; schemes offered by society to help people to translate the enigmatic messages coming from the other. But you must analyze these schemes of answers, and you find these schemes of answers in our society, but not necessarily in the society of the United States. In the USA, you have different myths than we have in Germany because you have another culture, another history, and so on. But for Laplanche, the myth is something you must analyze; it's not an answer for the problems we are dealing with.

BBT: One of the things you said is you do not necessarily find myths in metapsychology.

UH: Yes, you understand very well. You won't find myths in the metapsychology of Laplanche. At least that's what he's trying to do, not to use myths in metapsychology.

BBT: That raises two questions, and one is, why don't you think you will find a myth in metapsychology? The second is, Laplanche is very controversial. I don't know if you've had the experience, but oftentimes when people give presentations about Laplanche's work and stick very close to Laplanche, it creates a kind of irritation in the audience. I wonder about what this kind of focusing on metapsychology, taking out myths, stimulating, leaving something enigmatic, does.

UH: I understand this irritation. In my view, for Freud, the myth is a part of metapsychology. Look at the Oedipus complex, *Totem and Taboo, Moses and Monotheism*. These texts are quite difficult to understand if you don't accept that there is a part of mythology inside. How is it possible that we are talking about a time period spanning thousands of years and we want to find the origin of religion, for example, in *Moses and Monotheism*? I think Freud also has concepts in that text which, for Laplanche, are mythological, so I do not totally agree with what Laplanche is saying. Laplanche is the one in our society who insists the most on the scientificity of psychoanalysis, so he likes to exclude everything not scientifically demonstrable. Laplanche didn't talk much about books like *Moses and Monotheism* or *Totem and Taboo* because, for him, they're too mythological.

But you asked me why I think that the leaning-on theory has a mythological aspect, and my answer is that it's not scientific, which is easy to say. Where are your arguments? Perhaps you know that Laplanche excluded from his thinking the idea that the unconscious is inborn, that there is a genetic heritage in mankind; everything that doesn't come from the experience you have with others is excluded from his theory of the unconscious. Of course, there are experiences which are transmitted by society, but he calls this the mytho-symbolic, and he says the mytho-symbolic is always a kind of resistance against the discovery of the repressed. He says the mytho-symbolic is not the kernel/core of the unconscious. He disagrees with the reading of Lévi-Strauss and of Lacan, who structure the unconscious.

BBT: Returning to the clinical case: something that stood out to me in our discussion about it, which is something that others have also spoken about as well, was balance, and maintaining a balance in the tub.

Something you said was, "You learn more when you are outside of the tub; you will learn more from the unconscious of the patient." I was wondering if you could say a bit more about what you mean by that.

UH: I would say that you are in balance when the drives are not attacking you too much, and in my view, *le baquet* [the tub] is a metaphor for saying that you are capable of containing your drives. I think *le baquet* has to do with Freud's *The Interpretation of Dreams*, in the seventh chapter, where he speaks about the unconscious and consciousness. He describes a linear picture that goes from left to right. Then Laplanche took up a footnote from Freud where Freud says, perhaps we can make a circle, which is different from a linear psychic apparatus. These are my first associations for *le baquet*.

The tub tries to give a frame to all impulsions you have in your psychic apparatus. "Impulsions" is a word Freud uses in the beginning. I don't know if it's the same in English, but in German, you have two words: *Impuls* and *Trieb* [drive]. In French, you have *impulsion* [impulse] and *pulsion* [drive]. In Freud, you'll find *Impuls;* and later on, you will find the German word *Trieb* [drive], or in English, instinct; later on, the translation becomes drive. In French, they also began with instinct—you can find texts of Lacan's where he's talking about *l'instinct,* the French word for instincts; and later, they invented the word *pulsion,* and now everybody is talking about *pulsion* in French.

Le baquet is responsible for making sure that your impulsions and your drives are properly contained, so that you don't act them out by motility. I think that Laplanche created a new image, where the self-preservative side of our psyche and the sexual drives are combined. Let's start with the dream. In the dream, you can't move, your ability to move is cut, and the stimulation coming from outside is reduced to a minimum. What's going on is just the *Sexual*. I think *le baquet* comes from this idea that you can't move, and now the *Sexual* rises up. He takes *le baquet* as the model of the analytical treatment. It says, let's hear what the patient is saying about his unconscious, or about his sexual drives. That's my idea of *le baquet*, and that's why we say, don't act out, but stay inside *le baquet*.

Bibliography

Freud, S. (1958). *Totem and taboo*. Hogarth Press.

Freud, S. (2016). *Three essays on the theory of sexuality: The 1905 edition* (U. Kistner, Trans.). Verso.

Freud, S., & Jones, K. (1967). *Moses and monotheism*. Vintage Books.

Freud, S., Robertson, R., & Crick, J. (2008). *The interpretation of dreams*. Oxford University Press.

Hock, U. (2024). *Die rätselhaften Botschaften des Anderen*. Psychosozial-Verlag.

Laplanche, J. (1980a). *Problématiques I: L'angoisse*. PUF.

Laplanche, J. (1980b). *Problématiques II: Castration. Symbolisations*. PUF.

Laplanche, J. (1980c). *Problématiques III: La sublimation*. PUF.
Laplanche, J. (1998a). *Problématiques IV: L'inconscient et le ça*. PUF.
Laplanche, J. (1998b). *Problématiques V: Le baquet. Transcendance du transfert*. PUF.
Laplanche, J. (2011). *Freud and the sexual*. The Unconscious in Translation.
Laplanche, J. (2017). *Problématiques VII: Après-coup*. The Unconscious in Translation.
Laplanche, J., & Carson, L. (2007). *Hölderlin and the question of the father*. ELS Editions.
Laplanche, J., & House, J. (2016). *New foundations for psychoanalysis*. The Unconscious in Translation.
Laplanche, J., & Leclaire, S. (1972). *The unconscious: A psychoanalytic study* (P. Coleman, Trans.). *Yale French Studies, 48*, 118–175.
Laplanche, J., & Mehlman, J. (1976). *Life and death in psychoanalysis*. Johns Hopkins University Press.
Laplanche, J., & Mehlman, J. (2015). *Between seduction and inspiration: Man*. The Unconscious in Translation.
Laplanche, J. & Nicholson-Smith, D. (2015). *The temptation of biology: Freud's theories of sexuality*. The Unconscious in Translation.
Laplanche, J., & Pontalis, J.-B. (1965). *Fantasme originaire, fantasmes des origines, origines du fantasme* [Primal Fantasies]. Éditions des Grandes-Têtes-Molles de notre époque.
Laplanche, J., & Pontalis, J.-B. (1988). *The language of psychoanalysis*. Karnac Books and the Institute of Psychoanalysis.
Laplanche, J., & Pontalis, J.-B. (1988). *The language of psychoanalysis* (1st ed.). Routledge. https://doi.org/10.4324/9780429482243
Laplanche, J., & Thurston, L. (2020). *The unfinished Copernican revolution: Selected works, 1967–1992*. The Unconscious in Translation.
Scarfone, D. (2015). *The unpast: The actual unconscious*. The Unconscious in Translation.
Scarfone, D., Laplanche, J., Bonnigal-Katz, D., & Pontalis, J.-B. (2015). *Laplanche: An introduction*. The Unconscious in Translation.

3 Maria Teresa de Melo Carvalho

Universidade Federal de Minas Gerais, Minas Gerais, Brazil

Interview conducted in Portuguese and translated into English.

Maria Teresa de Melo Carvalho: I read the English version and the French version of this question and then I went on to think about it. When I wrote it down in Portuguese, I wrote down: "What is analysis according to Laplanche?" I was thinking from that question; when I had already thought about many things, I realized that the question was not exactly that. It was: "What constitutes a Laplanche *style* of psychoanalysis?" I don't remember which is the formulation in French, but it's something like "What is a Laplanchean analysis?" I thought, it's not the same thing, but I thought that from my point of view for someone to exercise an analysis according to a Laplanchean approach, he would first have to know what the conception of analysis is for Laplanche. A Laplanchean *style* of psychoanalysis must meet the Laplanchean conception of analysis, so I left my answer as I had thought.

Bryan Batista-Thomas: Okay.

MTMC: For me to follow a Laplanchean *style* of analysis, I would have to understand what the conception of analysis is for him. The word *style* like this poses a bit of a problem for me because the *style* I attribute to something very personal. Let's suppose that several of my colleagues think that they exercise psychoanalysis according to Laplanche's conception. But certainly, the styles of practice of each one will be very diverse. It is in this sense that I think that style is a very personal charac teristic of the analyst. I also thought that it would be necessary to have a preamble to an answer to this question: "What is Laplanche's conception of analysis?" The preamble is the following: I want to remind you that,

DOI: 10.4324/9781032670287-4

> for Laplanche, theory and the clinic go together. For him, there is not a theory of the clinic or a theory of technique independent of the theoretical conceptions that constitute metapsychology.

Freud conceived psychoanalysis as a method of investigation of the unconscious, a method of treatment founded on this investigation, and a theoretical body in which the data brought about by the methods of investigation and treatment are systematized. In this definition given by Freud, we see that these three levels indicate this cohesion between theory and the clinic. This is just a preamble to approach what I think would be Laplanche's conception of analysis.

There are a few texts of Laplanche's that deal directly with his conception of analysis to which I want to refer. These texts are from very different periods of his work since 1968. The first one was from 1968, entitled "Interpreting (with) Freud," in *The Unfinished Copernican Revolution*. Then there is *Problématique V: Le baquet: Transcendence du transfert* [The Tub: Transcendence of Transference], which is totally dedicated to this theme. These were courses that he lectured at the university from 1979 to 1984. A series of classes were then transcribed and published in *Problématique V*. Then there is a text on "The Interpretation between Determinism and Hermeneutics: A New Approach to the Problem (1991)" and the text on "Transference: Its Provocation by the Analyst (1992)," both in *The Unfinished Copernican Revolution*. The last one that I refer to is "Psychoanalysis and Psychotherapy (2006)" in *Freud and the* Sexual.

I think that in these texts, we can find the essentials of Laplanche's conception of analysis; then, I thought it would be interesting here to try to answer this question, "What is analysis for Laplanche?" by evoking in each of these titles something that is fundamental in his conception of analysis. The first one is "Interpreting (with) Freud": The title can be read in two ways because the "with" [*avec*] is in parentheses, so you can either read "Interpreting Freud," or "Interpreting with Freud," or it would be the idea "Interpreting Freud with Freud." The term "return on Freud" that Laplanche creates by modifying the term used by Lacan, "return to Freud," means that we need to return to Freud in order to read Freud and recover the Freudian discovery that would be misrepresented by post-Freudian psychoanalysis. Lacan called upon his students to do that. However, to show the difference in his position in relation to Lacan, Laplanche used this expression "return on Freud": To show the difference of his position and to mean that this "on Freud" has a sense of "not sparing Freud"—not sparing Freud because he is going to read Freud's text with a critical eye and with an analytical eye.

In fact, he will apply to Freud's text the method that Freud discovered for psychoanalysis, for the analytic treatment. The "Interpreting Freud" will demand a reading of Freud's text in which he would not look only for coherences, the evolution of the work as if Freud had started from a less evolved point to arrive at a more evolved point in the work. Then Freud's first writings would be outdated; this is not Laplanche's position. He thinks rather that psychoanalysis itself as a discipline does not progress by gradual achievements toward a happy ending—psychoanalysis progresses by going back to the sources. That's how he read and studied Freud's text. A text to be analyzed with an eye guided by the interpretive method created by Freud himself. This method does not aim at the manifest discourse. It does not aim at finding a latent meaning for the manifest discourse. From there comes the differentiation that he makes between a psychoanalytic interpretation and a hermeneutic interpretation. For Laplanche, psychoanalysis is not a hermeneutics. He discusses this at length in the essay "Psychoanalysis as Antihermeneutics" in *Between Seduction and Inspiration: Man*.

In this text, "Interpreting (with) Freud" (2006), he says what he thinks the psychoanalytic interpretation is, and that what characterizes the psychoanalytic interpretation is not the substitution of the manifest text for a latent text that the analyst could propose, based, for instance, on his own theory or on information that the patient has been providing. It would not be a construction in the sense of what Freud uses in the text *Constructions in Analysis* (1937). Interpretation is not equivalent to construction for Laplanche. Not that one cannot make constructions in an analysis—it is legitimate that in the analytical treatment there are constructions. However, Laplanche thinks that constructions are more the task of the analysand than of the analyst. The analyst is responsible for the interpretation that aims at decomposing the conscious discourse—dismantling the organization of this discourse and searching precisely for its incoherence, its gaps, its impasses, because these are the elements that can reveal the unconscious.

BBT: Do you think you could apply this to one of the vignettes?

MTMC: Considering the first vignette, you present us with a patient's report. In this first one, you don't introduce the analyst's intervention.

BBT: Right.

MTMC: I'm going to review the vignette from the moment that we read the following: "The analysand wonders to herself why the boyfriend made the decision for them to go there. She is partially irritated and feels that she cannot say no because it would be asserting a preference in the matter, which she has heretofore preferred not to do. She ends up attending the museum with her boyfriend." An analyst hearing this could propose an interpretation in the sense of hermeneutics, which is what Laplanche thinks is not the psychoanalytic interpretation. He could say, for example: "You thought about refusing, but you couldn't, because maybe this reminded you of previous experiences, even childhood experiences with your parents in which you couldn't assert yourself in the face of your parents' impositions, and this bothers you to this day." This would be a construction based on a theory that holds that adult behavior is grounded in childhood experiences—specifically at that moment in which the child would have that moment of self-affirmation before the limits of the other. The analyst could make this translation in a hermeneutic line.

Laplanche would not do this. Interpretation for him is a decomposition of the manifest content, where he would make remarks, highlight an element, and give greater weight to a certain element. For example, she says that she felt irritation, but she couldn't refuse it; then Laplanche could simply say: "You felt irritated…." A line like that gives weight on that part of the speech. "You felt irritated" emphasizes that speech within the speech. That sort of emphasis given on that part of the speech might cause the patient to talk more about her irritation. The person might go on: "Yes, I felt irritated; I thought this or that." This could bring more material that is latent, in the sense of unconscious, in this speech of hers. I use this example to illustrate the difference between what would be a hermeneutic interpretation and an interpretation in the psychoanalytic method, which Laplanche thinks is the legitimate one.

BBT: It's very close to Lacan to punctate speech in this way.

MTMC: Exactly! This text is from 1968. Laplanche was still relatively close to Lacanian conceptions. But regarding his conception of psychoanalytic interpretation, he remains close to Lacan's conception even after constructing his own theory. In a later text, *The Interpretation between Determinism and Hermeneutics: A New Approach to the Problem* (1992), he still holds to the same idea of what constitutes a psychoanalytic interpretation. By that point he had already developed his General Theory of Seduction, which was not yet present in this text from 1968. This will give him new elements to think about interpretation together with other elements that make up the analytic method for him, that make up an analysis. But you are right, interpretation as remarks, with the emphasis on an element, pointing out a lacuna, approaches the conception of interpretation according to Lacan, as Laplanche himself declares: ("[…]"interprétation": *deuten auf*, c'est indiquer du doigt ou des yeux; "pointer," pour reprendre ce terme au lacanisme." (Laplanche & Thurston, 2020, p. 412).[1]

The second text, *Le Baquet*, is the text about transference. What I want to comment on is this image that he uses to talk about the analytic space; he uses the image of a tub. It is a container, and in this image, he intends to materialize the idea that a container is necessary to create a potential difference between the inside and the outside. It is because he thinks that inside the analytic space, there should be the potentialization, the acceleration of the *pulsional* [drive], of the sexuality field. The analytic session makes a cut in the patient's daily life. He enters that space physically or metaphorically, when it is virtual, and leaves out daily life. It is the analyst who must attempt to preserve that space as a *pulsional* space. The analytic space is an installation, and the analyst is responsible for the maintenance of that space and for the attempt to always establish it as a place of the *pulsional*.

Laplanche gives a very simple example: The patient arrives to the session late and says, "Oh, I was delayed because of the subway strike. These strikes are disturbing our lives." The patient kind of starts a conversation with the analyst from a daily event that is disturbing his life. The analyst will hear that evidently; he will be able to answer, make some comment about the subway strike. He doesn't need to remain silent and neutral and let the patient's speech fall into a void. But he will be careful not to prolong it in a conversation that brings into the analytic space that which is of the order of interests. Laplanche calls this field the "self-preservation," using the Freudian term, or also using the expression "vital order," proposed by himself.

The distinction that he makes between self-preservation and sexuality is important here: The field of psychoanalysis is the field of sexuality, the *pulsional* field—not the field of self-preservation. That dualism that Freud initially established between self-preservation and sexuality, Laplanche thinks that, in fact, self-preservation and sexuality are not opposite poles in the *pulsional* field; they are two distinct fields of knowledge. Psychoanalysis, for him, happens entirely in the *pulsional* field. For Laplanche, the drive is always a *sexual* drive: *sexual* life drive and *sexual* death drive. The installation of the analytic space depends on the analyst's posture. It is up to him to protect that space as a space of *pulsional* circulation. It's up to the analyst to watch over the installation of that *pulsional* place and its maintenance. The analyst does this through what Laplanche calls *refusement:* It's a neologism in French (which in Portuguese would be *recusações*) to differentiate from denial, because denial is a defense mechanism.

BBT: Denial?

MTMC: Denial, yes. It's the analyst's *refusement* that helps to establish the place for the drive. These refusals are linked, to a degree, to what we call the analyst's neutrality. It is to restrain oneself in order not to respond from the point of view of vital interests, of the adaptive, the self-preservative. To remain attentive, not to respond from this point of view. There is also the notion of the refusal of knowledge. It's an appropriation that he makes from Lacan. But Laplanche will have a very particular conception of what Lacan called "refusal of knowledge." The analysand comes expecting the analyst to give him the solution to his suffering, to the questions that he brings, and the analyst doesn't have this solution. He does not know what constitutes his patient's well-being. He may even want the well-being of the patient, but he doesn't know what constitutes well-being for the patient. The analysand would put the analyst in the place of supposed knowledge, and the analyst refuses this place. He stays in the place of

> the guardian of enigma. This is the place that Laplanche attributes to the analyst—the guardian of enigma and pilot of the method. The analyst must guarantee the method of free association on the part of the patient. Give freely floating attention on his own part, and, at the same time, he is the guardian of enigma.

Besides that, the analyst is also the guarantor of the constancy of the framework. He must guarantee that constancy, the regularity of the sessions, and the duration of the sessions. Laplanche is against "logical time," for example. He thinks that there must be a regularity in the duration of the sessions and in the attitude of attention to the patient's speech. The analyst is not going to look at his cell phone during the session. He is not going to answer the phone when the phone is ringing. He is not going to read a letter as they said Lacan did. Things like this that are part of the analyst's attention guarantee the constancy of the analytic framework and allow the analyst to preserve the analytical space as a place for the circulation of the *pulsional* dimension.

In "Transference: Its Provocation by the Analyst (1992)," it is interesting to think that it is the analyst who provokes the transference. Laplanche recalls the proposition that it is the offer that creates the demand. It is the offer of analysis, the offer of the analyst, that creates not exactly analysis, but it creates the essential dimension of transference. That is why he talks about transference as a provocation by the analyst.

This transference is understood as the reopening of a relationship, as the reopening of the original relationship and structure of seduction. The analyst would be the analysand's other to whom the analysand addresses his questions, his enigmas—which were implanted in him by the adult world. The specificity of the analytic situation should be that of being able to circulate this *pulsional* that moves the patient's enigmas—these enigmas with which he was previously confronted during his constitution as subject. These enigmas impelled him to translations, impelled him to productions that left untranslated remains, and these remains continue impelling in search of new translations, answers. When addressing the analyst, the analysand is there, moved by his own questions, his own enigmas that challenge him again, and here the analyst is the guardian of enigma. The analyst does not have the answer. He will not translate for the analysand; he will provide for the analysand this possibility of translating again, of making a new translation for the questions that are there, propelling him from his origins.

The analysand arrives with his egoic discourse, with his ideologies or egologies; the analyst is there to open that, to make an opening in those constructions that in general are closed. They are limiting the patient's creativity, his life, and causing suffering. The analytic situation allows for de-translation and proposal of new translations. The analyst does not have the key to these new translations. He doesn't propose answers so that the subject can go back to questioning himself. The analysand can undo old constructions and translations to make new ones, which are less shut in, less committed to his defenses, less closed in a rigid ego.

In the essay "Interpretation between Determinism and Hermeneutics: A New Approach to the Problem (1991)," Laplanche speaks again of the differentiation in relation to hermeneutics, but he also speaks of the differentiation in relation to determinism since he speaks between determinism and hermeneutics. For him, there is indeed a psychic determinism, but this determinism does not have to do with an event, a raw fact. It is not a raw trauma that was inscribed there. There are facts, experiences of the child with the other, that can be traumatic, but there will always be a resignification, a translation of a first inscription of an enigmatic message. What will appear in the analysis is already a translation of something that was a message that was not only an experience that was registered and remembered just like this. Laplanche says childhood scenes are only interesting to psychoanalysis because of the messages they convey. In any childhood scene, if the patient is there remembering his story, the analyst must try to help him identify the message that this scene conveyed so that he can try a new translation for it.

For example, going back to the vignette of the analyzing woman who asks herself why her boyfriend decided to take her to the museum under these conditions. She felt irritated, but she couldn't refuse because that would mean asserting herself and setting limits, which she prefers to avoid. She then makes the visit. But it's interesting here that she takes it as a questioning. Why did her boyfriend decide to take her to the museum knowing that she didn't like museums very much, or else she just liked to go to the museum alone? He knew this information, but anyway he buys the tickets for them to go, and then this makes her wonder. When she poses this question, surely, she's looking for an answer, a translation for it, because she puts it as an enigma: Why did he do this to me? She is not saying that explicitly, but surely there is something latent behind this question that she is not able to formulate and that probably echoes original enigmas. From the point of view of the General Theory of Seduction, from the idea of the guardian of enigma and the reopening of the original seduction situation, it would be appropriate, upon hearing this speech, to say: "You wonder why he decided to take you." Put the emphasis and the accent on the question that stirs her up at that moment.

BBT: But in the irritation, also asking a question that causes the person to be interested in the other. "Why are you doing this to me?" "What do they want from me?"

MTMC: What does he want from me?

BBT: Yes, because the person's boyfriend is showing her something in this scene. What I am asking is in this situation, does the analyst ask something like this or does he simply keep this in mind: "What do they want from me?" "Why does she tell me this?"

MTMC: I think I understood. She asked this question, "Why did my boyfriend decide to take me to the museum anyway?" I'm saying, the analyst could reinforce that question: "Why did he do that?" When the analyst asks that question, he is looking for the translation that she has already made for that question. Because she has asked herself, "What does he want from me?" She asked herself, then the analyst is going to ask her what translation she gave to this question to which she found herself confronted by her boyfriend's attitude.

BBT: Got it.

MTMC: Her boyfriend's attitude triggered this question, this inquiry in her. Then she doesn't answer it here straight away, she could say: "Oh, I think he thought this and this." But no. Instead, she felt irritated, which is a sign that something of the *pulsional* is acting there. Some anger was triggered, and certainly this irritation has to do with a translation that she made that she is not speaking about because it is hard to say, or because she simply repressed it. If she has already repressed it, and she feels irritated, she doesn't deny her irritation, but she prefers to avoid confrontation. She has put herself in a conciliatory posture, an "egoic" posture of defense even against something that has taken over her there. It's OK that she didn't want to fight with her new boyfriend. That's not the only thing at issue: It seems that she didn't want to fight with herself, deal with a part of herself that would be there in action and that she didn't recognize or manage to put into her little story.

In the essay "Psychotherapy and Psychoanalysis," from *Freud and the* Sexual, Laplanche emphasizes the conception of analysis as a method of separation, of dissolution of the conscious discourse, thereby making it so that the lacunas, the lapses, can emerge working with interpretation. However, he also says that in a psychoanalysis, not everything is analysis. A large part of a psychoanalytic session functions as a psychotherapy in the sense that the analyst participates more actively, even in constructions for the analysand. (Laplanche distinguishes it clearly: Interpretation is the analyst's task; construction is left to the analysand. The reason is that the analysand already has the tendency to synthesize, which is to say, to make new translations from the new content that was enlightened by the analysis.)

Psychotherapy, however, is a process in which the analyst participates more actively, with measures of containment, with aids to constructions and translation. He functions exactly as a translational assistant. Laplanche speaks of the care that the analyst should have when the patient is psychotic or in serious borderline cases. In those cases, the method of analysis is not necessarily recommended, because where there is already a great deal of psychic disintegration, disconnection, one should not propose a method that disconnects, that analyzes, separates further. Laplanche says even in the analysis of a neurosis, the session takes place with many minutes of a process that resembles psychotherapy. The analysis itself is made up of privileged moments. Although, of course, all the time the analyst is going to put himself in the position of the guardian of enigma. The moments in which the analytic interpretation lights up unconscious content are rare moments during a session.

BBT: I'm going to take us back to something you said much earlier: you mentioned the term "subject" in reference to Laplanche's work. Do you know the development of the notion through his oeuvre?

MTMC: The term "subject" appears sometimes in Laplanche's texts, but certainly it is not a term that is part of the Laplanchean conceptual arsenal. On the contrary, Laplanche tends to avoid the term "subject" in the same way that he notes that Freud avoided it. During one of his *Journées internationales Jean Laplanche* [Jean Laplanche International Conferences], Laplanche said, when commenting on the term "subject," that Freud used it very rarely. He gives the example of the text "Instincts and Their Vicissitudes (1915)," in which Freud uses the term "subject" to talk about the opposition subject-object.

Laplanche also says that the movement of subjectivation is fundamental for the human being, but the "subject" is not found either at the beginning or at the end of this movement of subjectivation. Therefore, we see that he even (actually) avoids the term "subject." Laplanche also criticizes and systematically avoids the expression "subject of the unconscious," which was used by Lacan. He criticizes this expression in *Problématique IV* (1981) on page 124 in the French edition.

However, Laplanche considers it pertinent to speak of the "subject of self-preservation." What I'm going to quote is from a speech that he gave during a *Journées internationales Jean Laplanche* held in Spain, in 1999: "If we amplify the notion of subject to a center of action, eventually transitive and reciprocal, I see no reason not to talk about a subject of self-preservation." He admits that we can speak of a "subject of self-preservation" in this sense—that there would be a center of action that is eventually transitive and reciprocal, that interacts with the other. This is related to the fact that it is necessary to suppose an interaction or an early communication between the baby and the other. In the domain of the vital field, it is necessary to suppose an opening of the baby to the other so that the baby can be interpellated by the enigmatic message. It should be noted that it would be completely unreasonable to say that by agreeing with the expression "subject of self-preservation," Laplanche would be proposing a continuity between the "subject of self-preservation" and the process that will result in the constitution of the psychic apparatus as he conceives it. That is to say, the "subject" as psychoanalysis conceives it.

BBT: How does Laplanche's Translational Model of Repression represent a refusal of a psyche/body dichotomy? How does this refusal permeate through his work, like in the case of a radical failure of translation?

MTMC: I looked at this question and suggest a reformulation. I would rather ask: How does Laplanche treat the mind/body dualism in his theory, and in what way does his treatment of this dualism resonate with his Translational Model of Repression? Particularly considering the case of the radical failure of translation.

The soul-body or mind-body dualism is one of the oldest metaphysical questions. Laplanche said that psychoanalysis does not solve it. It instead displaces it to another dualism, which is the dualism between self-preservation and sexuality. He makes a transposition by considering the opposition between self-preservation and sexuality as two distinct fields of knowledge. On the two poles, whether on self-preservation or sexuality, there is both mind and body.

The newborn does not yet have his psychic apparatus constituted, in the psychoanalytic sense, but he already has a body and a mind. He perceives and registers traces of memory. The newborn is a body-mind unit. It is in this sense that Laplanche speaks—there is body and mind in the two poles: of self-preservation and sexuality.

I think that this way of approaching the dualism of body-mind has repercussions exactly in his refusal, for example, of the idea of the "amential unconscious" that was proposed by Christophe Dejours. I will read you a footnote of Laplanche's from *Freud and the* Sexual in the essay, "Three Meanings of the Term 'Unconscious' in the Framework of the General Theory of Seduction," when he's talking about why he doesn't accept the term "amential unconscious." But rather, he prefers the term "*enclaved* unconscious." He says that for him it is "difficult to accept, for it [the amential unconscious] presupposes that repression-translation is a process of mentalization which the psychotic unconscious does not undergo. It therefore presupposes that the messages of the other are not 'mental' but must become so. I have trouble accepting any such opposition as soul/body, *mens/soma*" (Laplanche, 2011, p. 218).

Now, I think it would be a good time to introduce the second clinical moment with the nosebleed. It is quite enigmatic, challenging, and in fact, it is difficult to analyze a fragment independently of the general context of the patient's analysis. However, I will take this bodily manifestation of the nosebleed to make some conjectures and considerations based first on the return of what was repressed and then on the radical failure of the translation.

The first question I asked myself was the following: Could we think of this bodily manifestation of a nosebleed as a hysterical symptom, in which the bleeding would have a symbolic character? That is, it would be symbolizing an unconscious content that would have been driven by the analyst's intervention? If our hypothesis is that of a hysterical bleeding, then it would be appropriate to seek the repressed element behind this conversion symptom, requesting the free associations of the patient. Then, following the method in which we work with symptoms, in the sense of the compromise formation, that is, the compromise between the unconscious content and the defense. Then, in this sense, the nosebleed would have a symbolic value because it is supposedly associated with an unconscious representative element, a residue of some translation that was made of a message from the other. The method of free association together with the analyst's interpretation could then bring to light the repressed content.

The other possibility would be: What the analyst knows of this patient suggests, on the contrary, that the bleeding appears as a bodily reaction to some *enclaved* content, according to Laplanche's terminology. Which is to say, it is related to an enigmatic message that would not have been translated. It remained there in the unconscious, stuck in the enclave, and for some reason it was reactivated in that session and its content's manifestation was bleeding. This nosebleed, body symptom, would be signaling the reactivation of messages that were never translated and that, therefore, did not leave unconscious remains. In this sense, bleeding would not be symbolizing anything, no other content.

If this is our hypothesis, that this bodily reaction was due to the *enclaved* unconscious that is somehow reactivated, then the analyst's intervention would be of another type. He should act as a translational assistant and not as someone who is going to ask for the patient's free associations. As a translational assistant, the analyst would propose a construction that seeks to translate the relation between what was said by the analyst and the patient's corporal response.

For example, perhaps the analyst could say: "It seems that you felt what I said was like a punch in the nose," which would be something along the lines of this second hypothesis. I would understand that the *enclaved* content is not just a bodily register. It is not a bodily reaction that repeats itself independent of a psychic register, but rather a register made at the same time of mind and body. The bodily memory of a bleed, for example, that occurred when the patient was confronted in his past with an injunction of the same type as the analyst's speech would have resurfaced. In this vignette, the speech of the analyst is quite superegoic, do you agree?

BBT: Yes.

MTMC: In some ways, the analyst is saying: How can you give yourself the right to pleasures if you do not fulfill your duties? It's in this sense that I said that the patient may have experienced this as a punch in the nose, a reprehension that was felt as something corporal. Even if the nosebleed does not symbolize the repressed content, it can be linked to a scene of seduction experienced in the past. That brings this element of a superegoic injunction, and the patient would not have been able to translate it, and it is then reactivated in this psychoanalytic session.

BBT: What are the ethics of a Laplanchean *style*? And how do they relate to metapsychology, clinical practice, and culture?

MTMC: When I read the word "ethics," it made me think of the essay "Responsibility and Response" in *Between Seduction and Inspiration: Man*. Laplanche starts from a curious question from Freud which is whether the patient is responsible, whether a person is responsible, for the unethical contents of his own dreams.

Laplanche starts from this and displaces the responsibility on the answer that the patient may give to enigma, those enigmas that constitute him. However, I remembered this text because at the end of it, he says that when he dislocates the responsibility on the answer, he did not want in any way to outline an ethics or a moral of psychoanalysis. Therefore, when he talks about responsibility and answer, he's not thinking about ethics in the general sense.

I think this is important to comment on because psychoanalysis does not propose to be a discipline that can deal with ethics in the general sense. This is a philosophical question that goes far beyond psychoanalysis. Now thinking about a regional ethics, let's say, within the conception of the analytic session, I think that what comes to mind is again the position of the analyst as the guardian of enigma, the one who doesn't know what is good for the patient. The patient comes asking for an answer from the analyst for his suffering. What could the analyst suggest to mitigate the analysand's suffering? The analyst doesn't know. Therefore, the only ethical position that he can have, according to the conception of psychoanalysis that Laplanche sustains, is that of the guardian of enigma. The analyst refuses to place himself in the place of supposed knowledge, as Lacan said. It is by refusing this place that he will provide the analysand with the re-encounter with his original enigmas and will help the patient to unleash this process of de-translation and re-translation of his original enigmas.

BBT: You spoke a little about how it relates to metapsychology and clinical practice. How about to culture?

MTMC: Maybe we can elaborate an answer starting from that text by Laplanche, "Sublimation and/or Inspiration" in *Between Seduction and Inspiration: Man*. That essay I think comes closest to this reflection, but I couldn't elaborate an answer. However, this bears some relation with the idea of the transcendence of transference, which is the end of an analysis in the Laplanchean perspective. The end of the analysis doesn't mean that the analysis is finite; it means that there is a moment in which the analyst realizes that the patient would have closed a cycle there. It is a propitious moment for the analysand to leave the analytic treatment and continue his analytic process in his relationship with the culture in general. This is the idea of the "transcendence of transference," which goes beyond the space of the analytic treatment.

The patient will be able to continue working from the reopening of his original enigmas in the face of cultural productions, for example, which is what Laplanche works on in this text, "Sublimation and/or Inspiration." Freud, when faced with Leonardo's work of art, asks himself something like: What kind of sublimation is this? Laplanche, in turn, wonders if this work of art would not be a privileged cultural production in the sense of allowing those who contemplate it to reopen their enigmas.

BBT: What parts of Laplanche's theory are lost when translated into a different culture and language?

MTMC: Laplanche was Freud's translator. As Freud's translator, he had a theory of interlingual translation. There are at least three of his texts where he talks about interlingual translation. Laplanche says the following: That in translation between two languages there are difficulties, but not failures of translation. While he uses the term "translation" in his theory, within his metapsychology, he is not making a passage from the field of the theory of interlingual translation to the translational theory of repression; there is no direct transferring from one to the other.

There are three essays where Laplanche takes up this issue: "Treating Freudian Translation (1984)," "The Wall and the Arcade (1988)," both in *The Unfinished Copernican Revolution*, and "Failures of Translation (2002)," in *Freud and the* Sexual. It's mainly in the "Failures of Translation" that Laplanche says that there are difficulties of translation, but he wouldn't talk about failures of interlingual translation. He would speak about the limits of interlingual translation. So mainly, for example, when it comes to translating the Freudian texts *Zur Psychopathologie des Alltagslebens* [*Psychopathology of Everyday Life*] (1901) and *Der Witz und seine Beziehung zum Unbewußten* [*Jokes and Their Relation to the Unconscious*] (1905), you can't do a translation and maintain the effect of the joke or the foul act. It's necessary to make a commentary. In the translation of Freud's book of jokes, when read in another language, you will find frequent footnotes. Because if you translate it literally, you lose the joke, the foul act. This is why Laplanche says these are not failures of translation but a limit of translation. When you translate a joke from German to English, it loses what makes it funny. These two Freudian texts are examples of texts that often require a commentary, but still, it's not a failure of translation, it's a limit of translation. However, with regard to the notion of translation in his Translational Model of Repression, Laplanche speaks of translation failures, failures that are inevitable due to the unconscious character of the enigmatic message, unconscious for the sender of the message himself.

If the translator has good theoretical support, that is, a consistent theory of translation, and has a deep knowledge of Freud's work, as in Laplanche's case, there should be no great losses in the passage from one language to another. I think that for the writings of Laplanche, we could think the same. If Laplanche is well translated, with a translator who knows his work and who is supported by a methodology and a theory of interlingual translation, he will be able to pass the theory into another language without significant losses. This is the ideal scenario, but we know that ideal scenarios are far from possible, so there are losses due to translational problems.

BBT: Did you notice any losses from French to Portuguese?

MTMC: I did notice translation errors.

BBT: Errors?

MTMC: Yes, I can give you examples of errors of translation in the book Sexual: *A sexualidade ampliada no sentido freudiano* [Sexual: *Expanded Sexuality in the Freudian Sense*] that was translated into Portuguese a few years ago. There are mistranslations. For example, they inverted the sense of the sentence on page 278: instead of "*nem mesmo é uma mensagem*" [it's not even a message], it says: "*é apenas uma mensagem*" [it's just a message]. Another example of an error of another kind, on page 118: instead of "*a tradução intralinguística não seria somente intralinguística [...]*" [intralinguistic translation would not only be intralinguistic], it says "*a introdução intralinguística não seria somente intralinguística [...]*" [intralinguistic introduction would not only be intralinguistic].

That's very serious. This is not a problem of being translated into another language. It is a problem of being mistranslated. Each essay of *Sexual* was reviewed by a Laplanche scholar, but unfortunately, people miss things that should not have been missed. There was no translation team that could discuss terminologies. Or that the review of an essay could have been done by more than one Laplanche scholar. If more than one reader could have read the translation that was done by a translator who is not a psychoanalyst, this could have improved the situation.

Unfortunately, mistakes were made in translation. This alters the author's thought. In an ideal scenario, I think that there would be little lost in the translation. But when there is no review team working together, or when there is no standardization of terminology or no attention to the same term that appears in various texts from different periods, the risk of mistranslation is great. The significant example that Laplanche gives us of this loss is in the translation of Freud into English. As a side note, Laplanche praised the work of Strachey. While Strachey was a great connoisseur of the Freudian work, and he was a good translator, he worked very much alone. He needed a team to help him there in the huge task that was translating Freud's work.

Strachey translated the term *Nachträglichkeit,* or *après-coup,* differently according to the context. Therefore, Strachey has at least two or three different translations for the same Freudian term ("deferred action," "subsequently," "later"). This made this Freudian term pass unnoticed as a conceptual notion ("*Faute, nous le verrons, d'une traduction adequate et d'une comprehension adequate, ou dirais-je, suffisament englobante, Strachey manque le concept*" (Laplanche, 2006b, p. 31)) [Lacking, as we shall see, an adequate translation and an adequate, or shall I say, sufficiently encompassing understanding, Strachey misses the concept.].

It seemed that it was simply a term of everyday language. Lacan was the first to realize that there was a constancy in Freud's usage of *Nachträglichkeit* that gives it a conceptual value, and then Laplanche, as Freud's translator who carefully read Freud's texts, confirmed this. This kind of loss happens and certainly may have happened in the translation of Laplanche into other languages. Some texts were translated into English, Italian, and German when Laplanche was still alive, and some of them, he was able to follow more closely, so he could oversee it. Laplanche's first translations in Brazil date back a long time, like the translation of *Problématiques I to V,* for example, and are, in general, quite good. I don't know if Laplanche followed them closely.

BBT: Do you notice a difference between the Laplancheans of Brazil and the Laplancheans of France or Spain or the United States, etc.?

MTMC: That's a little bit about what I was going to tell you now. This is related to the cultural dimension. Although France, Spain, the United States, in all these places where we know Laplanche was translated, we participate in this Western culture that shares several values and such. We have a very similar cultural soil, with specificities, of course, but very similar.

In Brazil, for example, psychoanalysis has a very strong influence from both English and French psychoanalysis. In the field of the humanities, the French influence in Brazil was very strong. We have a strong cultural identification with France. In fact, sometimes we have a reverence toward the colonizers, something that is currently being criticized.

I think there is a question that with the cultural reception of a work, it is important to ask: What interlocutors does Laplanche find in different countries? Who were the people, and from what disciplines are these people, who first received Laplanche? Let's take the United States for example.

BBT: Leo Bersani?

MTMC: Perhaps he could be an example; however, I thought about Jeffrey Mehlman, who was the translator of *Life and Death in Psychoanalysis*. This kind of interlocutor who is specialized in a particular field of the humanities and who is going to do the translation or the

> dissemination of the author's thought in his milieu is going to illuminate a part of the work that may go unnoticed for other Laplanche scholars. For example, Mehlman took *Life and Death in Psychoanalysis* as an example of a line within literary criticism. As if Freud's work was a literature and Laplanche was doing this reading of Freud's work according to a criterion, a method that could inspire a literary critic (Mehlman, in Laplanche et al., 1994, pp. 79–86). A scholar of Laplanche who comes from the area of psychoanalysis, more linked to psychology, would probably not think of this. This dialogue with this interlocutor comes from another area.

Then in the United States, also people interested in the study of gender went into dialogue with his work. This dialogue was what gave Laplanche the motivation to work on the concept of gender, which he had not yet worked on, so that the essay "Gender, Sex and the *Sexual*" in *Freud and the* Sexual is a discussion on this. Judith Butler, for example, has a reading of Laplanche. She uses Laplanche's theory to think about some specific questions of her research—a philosopher interested in these questions of gender. I think that the theory is being illuminated in different points by different interlocutors. There is another example that I think is very important. Silvia Bleichmar was a privileged interlocutor of Laplanche because she worked very closely with him, also doing her dissertation with him.

Silvia Bleichmar was an Argentine psychoanalyst who was exiled to Mexico during the military dictatorship in Argentina. When she was in Mexico, she did her doctorate with Laplanche. She didn't live in France. She did her doctorate at a distance, traveling back and forth. Bleichmar had a rich and lively clinic for children, and Laplanche was a psychoanalyst who never worked with children. He followed the work of Bleichmar and took great interest. She was a lively author, intelligent, and a questioning person. She made Laplanche confront several questions that concern the originary because he has his theory of the originary, but he never had children in the clinic as young as Silvia Bleichmar had. She would say: "I have patients that I see that the unconscious is not yet constituted there as a system." She needed a theory of the originary that would account for certain manifestations in the child's clinic and that questioned Laplanche's theory.

For example, Laplanche says: "The enigmatic messages of the adult are inscribed in the child's body." Then an author like her began to wonder: "How does this inscription take place? How can we describe it metapsychologically in a more precise way?" Also, the child translates the message, which is inscribed by the addressing from the adult and stays there in a state of waiting. In the *après-coup*, the child translates it and the rest that is not translated forms its unconscious. Bleichmar was one of the authors who asked: "But how can a little child that doesn't even have its psychic apparatus constituted translate or even receive an address from the adult as enigmatic? How is a little child going to interrogate itself from an addressing from the adult?" Then a whole discussion began to be created around the so-called "translator baby." Laplanche's interlocutors from different cultures confronted him with specific problems of their practice or specific problems of their culture. Another example: In Brazil today, there is a lot of concern in the university environment that does research on the issue of colonialism—to give a voice to the oppressed people here. There are already people who want answers to questions of racism—asking themselves, for example, would the designation of race be an enigmatic message parallel to the designation of gender? There is this kind of discussion that is starting to happen in academic circles among Laplanche scholars.

BBT: Do you think that the translation of Laplanche's work into German, Italian, Spanish, Portuguese, English, etc., contributed to change Laplanche's work? If so, in what way?

MTMC: I hope these translations have not contributed to changing Laplanche. Done well, they should maintain the integrity of his theory. But perhaps they could have made Laplanche's theory work in the same way he says he made Freud's text work, in the sense of what he himself defined as one of the aspects of his method of reading Freud.

I think that Laplanche seeks universality in his theory. The translation into a language other than French, in another cultural context, should not introduce modifications. Because within Laplanche's theory, he seeks something universal, valid for any human being in any culture. In this way, there could be no cultural relativism.

I agree with Laplanche when he states that psychoanalysis, like every scientific theory, has the universal and fundamental claim. Laplanche's proposition of the Fundamental Anthropological Situation seeks exactly to define a fundamental and universal situation of the origins of the unconscious, which is something that is independent of a specific social context. Laplanche's Translational Model of Repression would also be in the same place, that is, a valid model for any cultural context.

However, there is no doubt that particular social contexts have some influence at some point. I wonder where, in Laplanche's theory, what is relative to a specific cultural or social context would come into play. I understand that he places this relativity exactly in the ways of translating that are offered by the surrounding culture—what he calls the "mytho-symbolic." The mytho-symbolic is the entire cultural heritage that is available for a human being to translate their original enigmas. In this way, each cultural context will offer different forms of translation. For him, the mytho-symbolic is what brings this relativism.

I think that in cultures and societies different from the French one, with different languages, something that has a certain influence, not in modifying Laplanche's theory when it is translated, but it is again the interlocutors that he has in each place who illuminate one or another facet of his theory. Or those who criticize his theory and try to advance this theory, making it work.

Then, however, it is no longer Laplanche's theory as it was written and as it should be translated. It is Laplanche's theory already worked on and with the addition of that reader or translator who makes his own contribution.

Regarding the universality of the psychoanalytic theory, I am going to read a page here from *Between Seduction and Inspiration: Man*. It's the French edition, on page 305. Laplanche says: "In Freud's time we were certainly not postmodern. A scientific paradigm was not considered something to be arbitrarily chosen from a whole range of possibilities."[2] You can see that he is arguing that there is a psychoanalytic theory, a hardcore theory that cannot be negotiated.

There is also in this same collection a text that I think is very valuable for thinking about this, which is "Psychoanalysis: Myths and Theory." In this text, Laplanche places the entire universe of the mytho-symbolic in this place of cultural relativism. But the theory, metapsychology, the core of metapsychology would be universal. It should cross the diverse cultural contexts without alteration.

BBT: How does Laplanche's General Theory of Seduction and the Translational Hypothesis of Repression open a different perspective on the clinical vignettes?

MTMC: I spoke a little about this when I went back to a vignette you had proposed and considered the position of the analyst as guardian of enigma, and the analytic situation as a renewal of the confrontation between the analysand and his original enigmas. I think I can propose a vignette from my own clinical practice to accentuate a little more the perspective of the General Theory of Seduction.

The vignette is as follows: There is a nine-year-old boy whose parents came to me for consultation, with the complaint that their son was very undisciplined, challenging the limits at home, and showing indifference in schoolwork and in school.

In the initial interview with the parents, the mother gave me some examples of her son's indiscipline at home. His mother has seen him urinating in the potted plants and using his father's shaving cream and razor as if the boy were shaving himself, even though the boy had not gone through puberty.

In the first session with the child, I asked him to make a drawing of the theme he chose, a free drawing. He drew a girl. When I asked what he had drawn, he replied that it was a girl from his school whom he would like to date. The details that the mother brought, the girl in the drawing, among other elements of the case, can be taken as indicative elements of the pregnancy of this child's Oedipal experience, such as identification with the father, when he tries to shave like the father. Going further, there is defiance of the father's rules, as he recognizes that there is a prohibition, but even so, he defies it. There are indications of a choice of a love object when he is already thinking about his school sweetheart. Some elements, among many others, suggested this child's pregnancy of this Oedipal experience.

The boy and I talked a lot, using the graphic material as an intermediary for our sessions. In the third session, he was drawing when he suddenly asked me, "Are you married?" I took this question and the possibility of intervention and response, in the case of the analyst, to show the specificity of the Laplanchean approach. For example, if I were to intervene from a classical Freudian perspective, or even from a Kleinian perspective, I could have said something like, "I imagine you wish I wasn't married, because when you were younger and you found out that your mother was married to your father, you must have thought, 'What a pity that my mother cannot be only mine. Too bad she also must pay attention to my dad, and I can't have all her attention.'"

This would in no way be an intervention within the Laplanchean perspective, because this intervention proposes a hermeneutic interpretation. It would be the replacement of a manifest content by a supposedly latent content. The analyst imagines that the Oedipal scenario, the Oedipus Complex, is latent in the child's psyche. This intervention corresponds to an attempt to translate what would be latent in the child's psyche—trying to translate or symbolize what would be latent in the child's psyche when he asks me the question, "Are you married?"

What would be an intervention according to Laplanche's theory? Why does he explicitly criticize this type of intervention that proposes an Oedipal plot as an interpretation of something that the child is presenting, or even in the case of an adult? We need to remember that, for Laplanche, the analyst is the guardian of enigma. The analytic situation renews the patient's confrontation with his original enigmas. This renewal should move the analysand in search of new translations. It is not the analyst's task to propose a translation.

For example, it is not up to the analyst to propose a translation in terms of Oedipus. It would be better if the analyst remains someone who doesn't know about the patient's riddles. The one who will keep it, by placing himself as the guardian of enigma.

After the patient asked me, "Are you married?" I replied, "Why do you want to ask me that now?" Then the patient replied, "Because at your age, people tend to be divorced."

His answer surprised me a lot, and it opened a completely new perspective on my work with him. I understood that he seemed to be worried about his parents' possible divorce, because his parents were about my age. "At your age, people tend to be divorced." Since the parents were my age, would this kid be worried about the possibility of his parents separating? This opened a different path and this I understand to be Laplanche's perspective.

BBT: Given this difference that you've drawn, how would you compare Laplanche to classical and contemporary Freudian theory, Klein's theory, Bion's theory, self-psychology, and intersubjectivity, etc.?

MTMC: This example I gave is precisely to differentiate Laplanche's approach from a classic Freudian theory, in the sense of using Oedipus as the center of understanding the formation of neurotic symptoms. Klein's theory also places Oedipus very much at the center, although it takes Oedipus back to a very early moment. But she has many interventions based on the Oedipus Complex, on original fantasies, an arsenal of scenarios that Freud described as phylogenetic fantasies. Melanie Klein used this resource a lot for her interpretations. Freud mainly used Oedipus. It was a very apparent reading key in his clinical cases, mainly in the "Dora" and in the "Rat Man" cases. In the "Wolf Man" case also, from the perspective of the inverted, negative Oedipus.

I've studied self-psychology a lot, but nowadays I don't remember that much about that. I've studied the works of Heinz Kohut and Otto Kernberg, but mainly Heinz Kohut. He had a lot of influence here in Brazil in the late 1970s and early 1980s. It was a strong but fleeting influence.

One of the criticisms I make of self-psychology, basing myself on Laplanche's theory, is that the "Self" entered psychoanalysis as a way of rescuing the relationship between the "I" and "narcissism," which was undone by ego psychology. There is a whole debate between Hartmann and Kohut. Kohut is trying to rescue the "narcissism" that Hartmann had isolated from the "I." The criticism I make is that Kohut rescued narcissism, but at the same time, he separated narcissism from sexuality.

The "I" for ego psychology and for self-psychology has no immersion in the field of sexuality—it would be free from sexual conflict, it would have a sphere free of sexual conflict. While for Paul Federn, the author I studied for my dissertation, the ego (the I) is totally immersed in the libidinal field; it is constituted by the libidinal investment. Based on Laplanche, I could say that this occurs due to the other's libidinal investment in the child's body, which places the "I" entirely in the field of sexuality.

BBT: A difference I noticed, and I don't know if it's something cultural or about the people who studied with Laplanche. But the people I've interviewed in Brazil—you, Luiz Carlos Tarelho, and José Carlos Calich, and Lorenza Escardó in Spain—all of you talk about the Third Topographical Model. Now, the others I've spoken with, to my knowledge, do not speak about this model. I don't know if it's because they think it's a big change in Laplanche's work, a big influence from Christophe Dejours, and that the idea is more his than Laplanche's. That said, I noticed a huge difference in place, in culture.

MTMC: What you are bringing up is interesting. When we are discussing Laplanche, for example, outside the *Journées internationales Jean Laplanche*, or in the *Journées internationales Jean Laplanche*, when we are in an oral discussion, terms come up, and sometimes Laplanche himself used these terms when he was in an oral debate.

When we look in his written text, we don't find significant occurrences of the term "Third Topographical Model." It's funny because you get that term in your head, "Third Topographical Model," and one person says one thing and another says another thing, and you end up thinking you've already read the term in Laplanche. However, when you look for the text, where he would introduce the "Third Topographical Model," in "Three Meanings of the Term 'Unconscious' in the Framework of the General Theory of Seduction," in *Freud and the* Sexual, this term is not accentuated or emphasized.

Yes, we changed in that sense. On the one hand, it's a lack of rigor on our part in reading the author. I've even been paying more attention to it, because I'm writing entries for the *Vocabulaire de Laplanche*, which should be published in Fall 2024. I've seen myself doing that, putting a word, a term in my writing, and then I ask myself, did Laplanche use this term? Then, I'll look extensively through his writings, and many times I don't find the term I thought he had used. But, on the other hand, it is what I have already said, that is, the emphasis on a certain part of the theory or on certain terms depends a lot on the interlocutors we encounter in our context. As you noticed, in Brazil we have a big influence from Christophe Dejours, and some colleagues want to develop the idea of the Third Topographical Model that is originally his idea and not Laplanche's.

BBT: How does the reality of Laplanche's message and its materiality make Laplanche's theory a nonsubjective theory?

MTMC: I understand that the concept of message, with its reality and its materiality, shifts the foundational engine of the unconscious to the other, to another person—the person who addresses the child and whose enigmatic message will give rise to the unconscious. This other gives rise to the process of the constitution of the psyche. Not only the unconscious, but also the preconscious with what was translated.

This means that the little child, the newborn, does not have constituted subjectivity, much less the germ of subjectivity. He doesn't have something that is a becoming subject. For Laplanche, if there is no other with their addressing *to*, then the subject cannot be constituted. It is in this sense that I understand that Laplanche's theory is nonsubjective. The unconscious is completely desubjectivated; it is the realm of otherness, the otherness that has become internal otherness. It is the idea that the human being gravitates around the other; even though there is a closing movement, which Laplanche calls the Ptolemaic enclosure, he makes a contrast between Copernicanism and the Ptolemaic enclosure.

This movement must always, necessarily, go through the translation of the other's message. It is a movement of constitution of a place from where the subject will say "I." It contains translations of messages from the other. There is nothing there that came with the subject himself. There is no innate origin mark, no innate subjectivity, unless we are going to use the term "subject" to talk about the subject of self-preservation, in which case it is not the subject that psychoanalysis addresses.

BBT: Given that Laplanche did not study newborns and that his approach is not that of developmental psychology, how does his theory need and function with historical foundations? Bearing in mind both the clinical context of the analysand and their culture?

MTMC: I am not sure I understood the part of the question dealing with historical foundations.

BBT: Each patient has their own story. But this story, according to the example you gave about the boy, the enigma he has, something about seduction, has to do with parents and separation. I don't know what it would be, but there's a story there. Something foundational and concrete is present.

What I'm asking is that Laplanche didn't study newborns and his theory is not developmental in the psychological sense; it's developmental but not psychology. Therefore, how does his theory need and work with a person's history?

MTMC: He discusses this extensively in the text "Interpretation between Determinism and Hermeneutics: A New Approach to the Problem," in *The Unfinished Copernican Revolution*. It has a lot to do with that, where he places history, the historical facts of life. He takes a long look at the question of history itself, the way historians work. Then he comes to Freud with the case of Leonardo da Vinci, and then with the notion of *après-coup*.

That first deposit in the child's psyche is necessarily related to the other's message. It is not a story that registers raw facts. It is a record of an address from the other, and that will remain there waiting to be reactivated for another experience that makes an associative connection with that first one. In that connection, that first record is reactivated, and then, yes, there will be a translation.

What was lived will be resignified *a posteriori*. History is important, because precisely the child's history with his significant others, what he lived with these others, what was the address of these others to the child, what was marked or accentuated in the addresses of these others to the child, and what was deposited in the nascent psyche of the child will later, in the *après-coup*, be reactivated and translated.

It is in this sense that he says that psychoanalysis has a historical determinism, but history is understood in this process of *a posteriori* translation. It is not a determinism of raw facts, but it does not deny that events occurred that were registered in a privileged way in the child's psyche, and that they are always events that were examples of the address of the other—what was recorded as a message, because it was salient in the other's communication with the child.

BBT: This might be a rather strange question: Do you think enigma has a certain quantity, which is to say, there's a variation in the amount of enigma from something to a person? For example, let's assume that the *Mona Lisa* has a degree of enigma that's 90 percent. A person or child in front of the *Mona Lisa* is faced with this amount of enigma. While something else might have a 30 percent degree of enigma.

MTMC: Perhaps, we can relate this to Laplanche's text on inspiration and the idea of inspiration. Because there are privileged situations for reopening the original enigmas, one of these situations, according to Laplanche, is the analytic situation. It is conceived precisely to provide the patient with a reunion and confrontation with his original enigmas. It is a place where he goes to ask himself about his own things, he goes with the spirit of self-theorizing, of self-translating. If the analyst is in the position of guardian of enigma, this is a very favorable place for the analysand to face his enigmas, the enigmas that constituted him.

In addition, Laplanche said that there are cultural productions in front of which people also have the possibility of openness; they are inspired by the work of the other, that is, the work of the other makes them face their own enigmas and question themselves. I don't know if we could say that the *Mona Lisa* would be 90 percent enigmatic for all human beings—though she really is a masterpiece by a great artist—or if that is true for a portion of people and not for others.

It is not possible to say that other works or cultural phenomena would have more enigmas, would awaken more enigmas. We can think of the *Mona Lisa* because it is the figure of a woman with a half-smiling and half-not-smiling face, and this always refers to the question of the mother. The mother of a little baby. The look of the mother in relation to the baby. But what you're asking me about is inspiration. If there are situations that inspire more than others, in the sense that they would have a greater possibility of triggering or relaunching the questioning about themselves, about their own enigmas.

However, this would be a characteristic of cultural production itself, or of cultural production within a specific cultural context? Imagine a person who comes from the depths of Brazil, as we usually call it. A person who was raised in a rural area in Brazil, with little contact with works of art, who never heard of Mona Lisa. If this person is taken to see the *Mona Lisa*, we do not know if they will become either enchanted or inspired. I think there is a difference if that person sees the Mona Lisa in an art book that, by some chance, ended up in his hands, or if he is taken to the museum especially to see the Mona Lisa, by someone who tells him about the beauty, importance, and other attributes of this work of art. It also makes a difference if this other person who takes the person to the museum is a significant other for them, in such a way that the enigmatic "percentage" would be increased by the question: "What does this other person who takes me to the museum want from me? Why does he want me to see this work of art?"

It is in this sense that I say that we must ask ourselves if it's the cultural production itself that would be the source of inspiration, or if it is the cultural production in a cultural context, generally mediated by a personal context. In our example, it is necessary to consider the addressing of that other person who led the "uncultured" person, totally distanced from the world of art, to see such a masterpiece—if the person was inspired by the message of the one who led them or if it was the work of art itself that inspired them.

Notes

1 Trans. "[...] 'interpretation': *Deuten auf* means to indicate with a finger or a glance, to 'point,' as the Lacanians."

2 "There is a difference, to be sure, with the way things were in Freud's day. In those days, one was assuredly not 'postmodern.' A scientific 'paradigm' was not considered something to be chosen arbitrarily from an entire gamut of possibilities (Laplanche, 1999, p. 305)."

Bibliography

Freud, S. (1895). Project for a scientific psychology. In J. Strachey (Ed. & Trans.), *The standard edition of the complete psychological works of Sigmund Freud* (Vol. 1, pp. 295–397). Hogarth Press and the Institute of Psycho-Analysis.

Freud, S. (1896). Letter to W. Fliess of 6 December. In J. Strachey (Ed. & Trans.), SE (Vol. 1, pp. 233–239).

Freud, S. (1901). The psychopathology of everyday life: Forgetting, slips of the tongue, bungled actions, superstitions and errors. In J. Strachey (Ed. & Trans.), SE (Vol. 6, vii–296).

Freud, S. (1905). Jokes and their relation to the unconscious. In J. Strachey (Ed. & Trans.), SE (Vol. 8, 1–247).

Freud, S. (1915). Instincts and their vicissitudes. In J. Strachey (Ed. & Trans.), SE (Vol. 14, 109–140).

Freud, S. (1937). Constructions in analysis. In J. Strachey (Ed. & Trans.), SE (Vol. 23, 255–270).

Freud, S. (2016). *Three essays on the theory of sexuality: The 1905 edition* (U. Kistner, Trans.). Verso.

Laplanche, J. (1981). *Problématiques IV: L'inconscient et le ça*. PUF.

Laplanche, J. (1992a). *Transference: its provocation by the analyst*. In J. Fletcher (Ed.), *Essays on Otherness* (pp. 214–233). Routledge.

Laplanche, J. (1992b). Interpretation between determinism and hermeneutics: A restatement of the problem. *International Journal of Psychoanalysis, 73*(3), 429–445.

Laplanche, J. (1999). Entre séduction et inspiration: l'homme. PUF.

Laplanche, J. (2006a). Interpreting (with) Freud. *Psychoanalysis, Culture & Society, 11*(2), 171–184. https://doi.org/10.1057/palgrave.pcs.2100077

Laplanche, J. (2006b). *Problématiques VI: L'après-coup*. PUF.
Laplanche, J. (2008). *La révolution Copernicienne inachevée: Travaux 1965–1992*. Quadrige/PUF.
Laplanche, J. (2011). *Freud and the sexual*. The Unconscious in Translation.
Laplanche, J. (2015a). *Problématiques V: Le baquet. Transcendance du transfert*. PUF.
Laplanche, J. (2015b). *Sexual: A sexualidade ampliada no sentido freudiano 2000–2006*. Dublinense.
Laplanche, J., & House, J. (2016). *New foundations for psychoanalysis*. The Unconscious in Translation.
Laplanche, J., & Mehlman, J. (1976). *Life and death in psychoanalysis*. Johns Hopkins University Press.
Laplanche, J., & Mehlman, J. (2015). *Between seduction and inspiration: Man*. The Unconscious in Translation.
Laplanche, J., & Thurston, L. (2020). *The unfinished Copernican revolution: Selected works, 1967–1992*. The Unconscious in Translation.
Mehlman, J. (1994). Verweile doch! Pour l'étayage. In J. Laplanche et al., (Eds.), *Colloque international de psychanalyse: Nouveaux fondements pour la psychanalyse – actes du colloque de Montréal (3–5 juillet 1992)*. PUF.

4 Dominique Scarfone

Canadian Psychoanalytic Society and Institute (Montréal French Branch), Montréal, Canada

Bryan Batista-Thomas: What constitutes a Laplanchean style of psychoanalysis?

Dominique Scarfone: Well, I'd say there is no Laplanchean style of psychoanalysis. Laplanche followed Freud's method—perhaps radicalizing it. In his theoretical practice, he used it in reading Freud critically, for instance, discussing the points where Freud has some second thoughts, hesitations; where he goes astray; and where he contradicts himself. Laplanche equated these points as the equivalent, though not the same thing, as slips and parapraxes or failed actions in a patient.

In his clinical practice, of which he never spoke, I guess that Laplanche had his own personal style of analysis, but there is no reason for any other analyst who is inspired by Laplanche to adopt a Laplanchean style. Just as Laplanche had his personal style, each of us can have our own, all the while heeding the Laplanchean lesson about what it is to work with the unconscious, to work with his conception of it.

Laplanche never taught any special "Laplanchean technique" or "Laplanchean way" of doing analysis. Laplanche mainly invokes the classic Freudian method, which allows each of us to go on being very personal and creative in our way of doing analysis, certainly inspired and guided by Laplanche's main ideas about the analytic setting and the analytic process. I am thinking mainly here of the "refusals" advocated by Laplanche, which, by the way, are inspired by Freud himself, who recommended that the analyst in the session should let go of any practical goal, any "purposive representation" regarding what he's doing, where he should go, or where the patient should go. Laplanche, again, mainly radicalizes this Freudian precept; he uses it in a more stringent way by demanding that the analyst refuses to even know in order to really present as freely as possible his mind as a receptor of what the

DOI: 10.4324/9781032670287-5

patient brings. Also, to not guide the patient to any pre-established ideological goals, like, for example, "assuming castration" in Lacan or "reaching the genital phase" with Freud.

BBT: How does Laplanche's Translational Model of Repression represent a refusal of a psyche/body dichotomy? How does this refusal permeate through his work, like in the case of a radical failure of translation?

DS: Very interesting question. I think that here is an opportunity to clarify something which is not always clear among those who read Laplanche. For Laplanche, every individual is always already a body-mind—a bio-psychological individual. Laplanche never separates the psychological—and I use psychological, not psychic, at this point on purpose—from the biological. The psychological is but a version, an aspect of the inborn bio-psychological entity that we are. (To clarify: Following Laplanche, the Freudian psychic apparatus, on the contrary, is not inborn; it results from the differentiation brought about by the translation/repression of the compromised messages.) For instance, when Laplanche highlighted *Anlehnung* in Freud's thinking [leaning-on, i.e., Strachey's *anaclisis*], his readers often interpreted it as the mind leaning on the body. For Laplanche, that's not at all what leaning-on is about. *Anlehnung* strictly refers to the *Sexual* domain leaning on the self-preservative domain. As we know, Laplanche later criticized this aspect of Freud's theory. Nevertheless, even as he criticized it, he found it necessary to remind us that it's never the mind basing itself on the body in a "leaning-on" relationship. We could rather say that the *Sexual* "leans on," or, better, "happens" as disruption in the bio-psychological, self-preservative domain.

Now, interestingly, you ask this in relation to the question of the Translational Model, which I think is an important question to ask. When we think of translation, we are immediately carried over to the side of the pure mind, the spiritual, the intellect, and so on. I think that this is also very possibly a misreading of Laplanche. For him, the message—that is, the contaminated or the compromised message from the adult to the infant—is not necessarily a verbal message. It is not necessarily loaded with intellectual or cognitive content. It can be a mere gesture. It can be touching. It can be an exclamation. It can be anything nonverbal, and therefore it is loaded with affect, with bodily elements, and so on.

This brought me to personally question the word "translation" itself. Because with the term "translation," we may easily lose sight of the fact that I just mentioned—that it's not about translating a text. I therefore prefer the word "transduction," because it designates a wider field, if you will, which includes translation, be it inter-linguistic or inter-semiotic translation. It's a wider concept because "transduction" can happen at many levels. For instance, our phones constantly do transduction from electromagnetic waves to sound waves and vice versa. Transduction implies a change of category. This is precisely what happens in seduction. What the mother does to the child, even her silence for that matter, impacts the child's mind without necessarily carrying a ready-made semantic content to be translated in the traditional sense. The mother's action must be transduced, the child necessarily trying to make sense of whatever it perceives from the adult world. I think that transduction would represent better what Laplanche had in mind.

The rejection of the body-mind dichotomy is present throughout Laplanche's work. Which brings me to your question about a radical failure of translation. The idea of a radical failure of translation must be examined closely. There is always translation, or, in my vocabulary, always "transduction," carried out; and the word "failure" merely means that the psyche—the translational psyche—never achieves a full transposition of the energy of the message into the energy of the translated result. There is always a remnant, always a residue, and this is what the failure in question is about. We sometimes speak, carelessly, of the infant's successful translations, which can be heard mistakenly as, "He got it right." But this is not what is meant by a successful translation. What it means is that the translational apparatus succeeded in creating meaning. Now, it's never said that the meaning is the adequate or "correct" meaning—the meaning that the adult intended, for instance. A correct meaning can be described at the cognitive level. For instance, "Here's how to hold your spoon, my little child, for eating your cereal." In such a case, there is indeed a successful, correct understanding of the manifest content of the message. What we, psychoanalysts, are interested in is the sexual dimension. The sexual stowaway, so to speak, within the message from the adult. There is a translation that works for the child's need to make sense, and we know that this making sense can be totally imaginary and factually wrong. Wrong or right doesn't matter, because every translated result shall be reviewed, revised, and updated time and again. This is what the "successful" in successful translation means—creating a meaning that for some time organizes the psyche, stabilizes the energies, and creates a form that can go on evolving.

I therefore don't think there is such a thing as a radical failure of translation. There is always translation and always failure. Now, I can imagine a situation where confusion is brought to the mind of the child in his or her effort to translate because of the superimposed, overly violent context in which the messages are emitted. That there is a confusing sort of translation on the part of the child, when the child tries to, at the same time, create meaning and comply with the meaning that is imposed by the other. But this is as close as I would get to the notion of a radical failure of translation.

BBT: Related to the previous question, in the refusal of the internal and external, where for Laplanche the external other becomes the internal other, what are the implications for clinical practice? For example, how does the analyst understand the session and/or the analysand's material?

DS: Here again, let me question your question. I don't think Laplanche would agree that the external other becomes the internal other. All the same, I think I see what your question aims at. What becomes internal is the *otherness*, which is not the same thing.

BBT: Can you highlight the difference, and how you understand "other" versus "otherness"?

DS: In non-Laplanchean analysis, there is this notion of internalization of the object relation, where the object is internalized and it becomes part of the subject. This is not how Laplanche theorizes things. What matters is rather that in the process of "transduction" or "translation," the residue, the untranslatable residue, the packet of energy that the child's psyche could not really deal with, stays there as a permanent internal irritant. It's an internal irritant, but one which is felt as external, as other, as foreign, by the child's psyche. Therefore, it's described as internal by us, the observers, who state that the subject and we all are dealing with an irritant which stems from within. However, it's always experienced as foreign; and this, incidentally, is why it lends itself so well to projection, whose purpose is of positing again a material external source.

It's the *otherness* of this irritant, which is internal, or better, internal/external. However, let me remind you that for Laplanche, we must beware not to replace the ego-centeredness of late Freudian theory with an id-centeredness. We are radically de-centered, so that the id or the repressed unconscious is not our new center. Indeed, there is no new center. We are always deported, driven astray by *otherness*. The *otherness* designates the radical "*strangerness*" of the "unconscious thing," if you will, whether it is within us or in the people we meet. Laplanche was therefore wary of not replacing the Ptolemaic ego- or self-centeredness of the late Freudian theory (or in some contemporary versions of psychoanalysis), with the idea that our center is the unconscious. For him, we are constantly and radically de-centered—always adrift, so to speak, in terms of a center. I think that this is interesting and important also clinically, because this should, for one thing, prevent us from looking for the "right" translation. Otherwise, the centeredness leads us back to the idea that we know where we should be going during the analytic exploration. Whereas this drifting, this radical de-centeredness, means that we really don't know. The refusal to know is not some posture we adopt. We are called upon to acknowledge that we really don't know. What we know is a few things about how the mind works, how translation works, how repression works, and so on. But always leaving it as much as possible to the analysand to do their transduction/translation.

As you know, in *Freud and the Sexual* (2011), there is a paper by Laplanche, "Psychoanalysis and Psychotherapy," in which he says the translator is mainly the patient. However, he acknowledges that sometimes, and perhaps more frequently than we would like, the analyst needs to intervene and to assist the patient's translation, and therefore to inject some meaning. I think this is unavoidable, because even our silence can easily suggest that we are of this or that opinion on what the patient is communicating. There is no pure analytic stance. But we should strive as much as possible to leave it to the patient to find their meaning, knowing that there is no final point of arrival. I think this is very radical in Laplanche.

For what regards understanding the analytic material, here again, the radicalness of Laplanche, I would say, is that we should resist understanding. Our job is not to understand; our job is to listen, which is not the same thing. Do not strive for understanding the patient, which would mean that the analyst is doing their own translation, whereas their role is to de-translate. We hope, of course, that in the end, we will arrive at a certain understanding that fits the analysand well in the sense that it can create a certain degree of coherence or cohesiveness of his psyche, in an evolutive form, that allows them to go ahead with their life.

But the analyst is there to point to what cannot be understood, to the misunderstandings. This was Laplanche's notion of interpretation—highlighting something the patient said. Pointing a finger at something that was mentioned without necessarily thinking that you are understanding anything. It's a kind of directing the spotlight on something that doesn't seem to fit in the intentional communication by the patient. "What will you do about it?" This questioning would be, ideally, the only role the analyst would play. But as I said, it doesn't always function in that manner. We are called upon to intervene and to inject some meaning. Otherwise, we are leaving the patient in such a state that he cannot really make use of our listening.

What do we understand about the session? I think that in the Laplanchean radical view, the analyst is the guardian of the frame (and guardian of "the enigma," but we have addressed this aspect with the refusal to know). What matters is to be able to ignore the self-preservative aspects as much as possible during the session so that the attention is turned toward the sexual dimension. I think that Laplanche's paper "Transference: Its Provocation by the Analyst," in *The Unfinished Copernican Revolution*, illustrates his clinical conception clearly. He never used a clinical example, and you don't need one. I think that every analyst who is working in the Freudian spirit of the method of analysis will readily see what Laplanche is pointing at regarding transference, the role of the frame, and the role of seduction operated by the analytic setting on the patient. I think it's clinically quite limpid, so that you don't need a clinical vignette. I would say that any clinical vignette you try to use will distort the matter to some point. Because, as I said in answering the first question, every analyst has their own style and therefore the vignette we give will always be biased, I would say, by our personal style and not necessarily usable by another analyst.

We *can* illustrate our ideas clinically. I published a paper in 2022 where I used an extensive clinical case, but it was to illustrate a totally different point. It's not about my method of doing an analysis because it's something I described. Something that happened against my best intentions. It was a very serendipitous event which proved useful. Because I totally did not understand what was going on. A patient two or three years after the end of the analysis wrote a letter to me where she was correcting my view of her analysis, which I had presented in another paper, and said, "I don't even remember what you're talking about. Here is what really mattered for me." She points to something else.

BBT: She read your paper of you writing up a case of her?

DS: Yes. I had given a paper at a conference, and it was published in a multi-authored book. My patient, who at the time had terminated her analysis, saw my name on the cover of the book. She was curious and discovered that I was speaking of a dream of hers in the paper. I thought that this dream had been pivotal in her analysis. She wrote me a long letter to say, "I don't think this was so important. Here is what was important." She gave me a lesson, which I am still learning from. Would I say I am finally understanding? Probably not. But I am certainly having a new understanding of her analysis.

Her version of the story has to do with Laplanche in the sense that what she found important is that for two or three weeks she remained totally silent for the whole session, and that rather than interpreting her silence, I, too, remained totally silent, patiently waiting until she emerged from her silence. I had forgotten about this event, but in her letter, she told me this was the most important thing in the many years of her analysis. I allowed her, she said, to be free and to come back to the surface, so to speak, by her own will. This was really a radical change in my understanding: The silence on my part meant that I really did not pretend or even try to "know" better than herself what was going on. It refers to Laplanche indirectly, of course. But note that this example is not my way of illustrating a theory, if you see what I mean. It is the patient who has taught me something.

BBT: That's very interesting.

DS: When you ask, "What are the ethics of a Laplanchean style?", having said what I said, I think that the ethics is there. It's the ethics of seduction. It's the ethics of knowing that the analytic setting and the analyst's desire—Laplanche would not want me to use this term; he was very critical of the word "desire," but let's use the word "desire," why not?—that the analyst's desire is seductive no matter what, and therefore, that the setting we put in place is seductive in the general sense of the word. Therefore, it entails an ethics of what I just described, of not knowing. Otherwise, we are doubling down on the seduction. When we intervene with our knowledge, we think we are clarifying things. In fact, we are confusing things a bit more because we are against our will, and without knowing it, we are again being seductive with our knowledgeable stance. We are then suggesting that we are in possession of a meaning that we can give the patient or deprive them of. We are thus intensifying the process of seduction. Actively refusing to know is the counterweight, the necessary counterweight to the seductive effects of the analytic stance, of the analytic setting, and of the analyst's desire to do the analysis.

BBT: I'm a little curious about this double seduction that you're mentioning because it almost sounds like it's a seduction of the context versus a seduction by the person. Is that safe to say, or how would you further elaborate on the double seduction piece?

DS: I wouldn't say that there is a seduction *of* the context. I think that the setting is seductive, but the setting is put in place by the analyst. Therefore, I refer to the analyst's desire. By putting a sign on my door saying, "Scarfone: Psychoanalyst," I am expressing my desire, my readiness to do an analysis. Therefore, when a patient finds my card or my door plate and comes and asks for analysis, this means that the offer precedes the demand for analysis. It's always the analyst, the person of the analyst, with their desire to do analysis, who is the seductive agent. Hence, it's not the setting as such that does the seduction. The setting is the extension of the analyst.

This means it's very difficult to do pure analysis. Actually, to try to achieve pure analysis would be, I think, crazy. The analyst will always be exerting a seduction, no matter what. But we must be aware of that and always re-invite, or reignite, in the patient the sense that they are the ones who should come up with their own interpretations, though knowing, again, that it's not totally possible. We are always working somewhere between a certain conception of "pure analysis" and, at the other end of the spectrum, the naive approach of therapists who think that they will have an ordinary conversation and explain things to their patient. We operate somewhere between these two extremes and should be constantly aware of the seductive effect of the analyst and aware of the possibility that whatever we do or say, or don't say, can still induce a certain seduction in the patient. Therefore, we must constantly travel to and fro between this objective effect of our presence and of our method (i.e., reopening the scene of primal seduction) and the assistance we can offer our patient to deal with it.

Let me stress again that Laplanche's Translational Model does not mean that the analyst is the translator. Far from it. The sole translator, ideally, should be the patient. Therefore, the ethics in Laplanche's model result not from his style, but from the core of the General Theory of Seduction, which entails that translation is left to the analysand.

Now, you ask how this relates to culture. I think it's a very interesting question, and what I am going to say would possibly make Laplanche turn in his grave, because I will mention Winnicott. Laplanche didn't have a high opinion of Winnicott, as I was brought to learn. I think that in spite of a different vocabulary and of a different theoretical framework, the issue that Winnicott addressed with the transitional space or the space for cultural experience resonates with the ethics resulting from Laplanche's General Theory of Seduction. About the transitional space or phenomenon, Winnicott says that we do not ask the child, "Did you find it there or did you create it?" There is a vast literature on the found/created paradox, but, to me, the main point here is that *we do not ask*, that we leave it to the child to freely think and feel whatever it thinks and feels. We are not forcing upon the child an answer, a cognitive formulation. We let a creative experience be. Winnicott also called the transitional space the locus of the cultural experience. In Laplanchean terms, in that locus we are dealing with the enigmatic, hence with the seductive aspect, with the untranslatable core of the experience. We can formulate many secondary ideas about our experience. But the experience itself is not translatable. It's not speakable. It's something that is not addressed to us, was not addressed to us intentionally. But when we are in front of a work of art, we feel that it "speaks to us," don't we? We often use this expression. The work of art is not speaking, of course, but it elicits in us a response, a response that is ours alone. We are not required to give a rational account of why we are so enthralled with this or that painting or sculpture or whatever.

This, in my view, is totally congruent with the ethics of seduction in Laplanche's model, where the patient is the translator.

BBT: How does this relate to Laplanche's conception of inspiration?

DS: Thank you for reminding me of this aspect. It has indeed to do with inspiration, in the sense that inspiration is, we could say, the cultural version of seduction. It's something that elicits in us an effort to give a response to a question that we cannot possibly formulate in words. But it inspires us in the sense that it entices the translational (or transductive) function in us. Here again is why transduction seems to me a more appropriate word. For instance, a painter in the twenty-first century who is inspired by a painting by Leonardo will start doing a painting of his own. Is that a translation of Leonardo's "message"? I don't think so. It's really transporting into another medium something that doesn't travel through words. It travels through a sensuous experience, and it gives way to a response which can be of many forms. A writer will write a text. A poet will write a poem and so on. These are all responses inspired by the message in Leonardo's work, but we see that the word "translation" is rather inappropriate because there is no precise meaning requiring translation. There is some wave of energy that elicits new forms in those who respond to it.

Think now of transference. The patient is carrying the irritant in himself that *transduces* into a transferential move. Was it addressed to the analyst from the beginning? Not necessarily. It could have transferred onto whomever the analysand met. During the analytic session, the analyst is there, in that moment, in that room, at the receiving end. But the material transferred was not necessarily originally meant for him or her. We analysts *interpose ourselves* as the receptors of the transference; it is a transference which we have provoked, but we have provoked it as a non-specific motion. We then receive something that was not initially meant for us. We are inserting ourselves in the trajectory of that motion, therefore we are creating an address which, I would say, gives the experience a more humane aspect, a more culturally significant aspect. This, of course, transforms in and of itself the experience in question by inserting it into the universe of meaning—a meaning that, from that point on, can be eventually articulated and even shared.

Our insertion in the trajectory also reflects the artificiality of the analytic encounter. This is not a natural situation; we created it from scratch by announcing that we are analysts. By creating an address, and by enhancing the intensity of the experience through the refusal to know and the marginalization of the self-preservative aspects and so on, we create what Laplanche called "the tub," where the intensity of the experience is brought to a high temperature, so to speak, which allows for de-translation and gives the analysand an opportunity to operate a different translation. The patient can thus fall back on a new, more meaningful symbolization; most importantly, a symbolization more open to evolution, to re-symbolization, whenever life demands it.

BBT: Which parts of Laplanchean theory are lost in translation into a different culture and language?

DS: I don't know, because I'm in the culture that I'm in. My speculation would be that not much should be lost, because Laplanche is looking at universal mechanisms. Whatever your culture or language, you are always translating (transducing). Though Laplanche doesn't speak of it in these terms, to me, transduction/translation is a fundamental function of the psyche. The psyche evolved always in the direction of better transduction/translation, for the sake of making sense, of creating meaning. Contemporary neuroscientists subscribe to this idea that the brain is evolutionarily directed at making sense of the environment, the human environment in our case, and therefore to make the individual better able to survive.

If indeed this function of creating meaning is universal, then I don't think that there is much to be lost in Laplanche's theory. We could discuss how the sexual is understood in different cultures. But there again, the sexual in Laplanche is not the set of behaviors we call *sexuality*, which can, of course, vary culturally.

BBT: You had spoken a little earlier about the violence of the context and its impact on the constitution of the psyche. I was hoping we would be able to speak a little bit more about that.

DS: The notion of translational failure would rest on the idea that there is a state or a context that is extremely violent and impedes, to a certain extent, the spontaneous process of translation. This of course refers to Laplanche's notion of intromission that forces the child to comply to what he perceives as the expected translation that comes from the violent parent. Therefore, there is a clash in the child's mind between what would be his personal translations.

My view of intromission is that the child's personal effort at translation clashes with the expectation that it senses in the violent other; an other that forces the acceptance of, let's call them, ready-made translations. This to me, as you know, resonates well with Piera Aulagnier's concept of secondary violence. I think that secondary violence in Aulagnier and intromission in Laplanche are equivalent concepts. At least, they go together very well. The result in both cases is a confusion and a radical conflict in the child's mind. More than a conflict, it is what Jean-François Lyotard calls a *differend*, which is a conflict where there is no possible resolution because there's no possible meeting of the contraries in order to form a compromise or to arrive at a shared verdict. You have a split mind, in a way. This is a deleterious form of the failure of translation. It's a failure in establishing cohesive or coherent sets of translations for himself that give the subject a certain sense of meaningfulness.

We must always be reminded that every translation leaves behind an untranslated residue. In that sense, as already mentioned, every translation is partly failed. As for the violence, we see that it is not necessarily in the message itself. The message can be, unconsciously on the part of the adult, affected by the same set of fantasies in the violent other as in the "ordinary" other. For example, the unconscious fantasy "I penetrate you." The different outcome depends on whether the transmission of the message occurs in a context where the child's freedom of translation exists or not; whether the child is, or not, bothered by a supplementary exigency, a supplementary demand on the part of the adult to comply to this or that way of understanding. The violence of intromission, therefore, does not rest on the kind of fantasies unconsciously entertained by the adult. It's more on how the child is treated in the relationship and, therefore, how free the child is to craft their own translations. In short, it's a question of whether the child is allowed to think for himself or not. It's the context, the violent handling of the child by the adult, that makes it an intromission rather than an implantation. This is not exactly what Laplanche says, but I think it is compatible with what he writes in his short paper on "Implantation, Intromission," in *The Unfinished Copernican Revolution*—that intromission impedes psychic differentiation in the child's mind, that is, the topographical differentiation; psychic processes are arrested due to the forced translation imposed on the child.

BBT: Something else that I would like to return to and see if you could elaborate a little bit further on is the id not being the new center as compared to the id being the center and there being no point of arrival.

DS: This is in Laplanche's book *New Foundations for Psychoanalysis*, where he warns us against not replacing the ego-centeredness with an id-centeredness. The unconscious, says Laplanche, is not really *my* unconscious—it's *in* me, but not mine; it's not *of* me, hence it is not my center. The de-centering is radical in the sense that if we were to posit the unconscious as our center, we would be negating what Laplanche calls its "strangerness" and would be entitled to try and find where it stands, what it is, and how it works in us, in order to domesticate it; whereas we don't know these things; we know only of the interference, the deviation the unconscious imposes on our thought processes.

The question is important for theoretical, but also for practical, reasons, in the sense that we run contrary to a certain formulation in Freud's earlier work, for instance, where it was a matter of "making the unconscious conscious." Whereas, here, we are not transforming the unconscious. Laplanche had a nice metaphor about this when he said that psychoanalysis is comparable to astronomy. That is, you can have a science called astronomy, but you will not change the stars, the heavens. You can describe the universe with mathematical equations, even make predictions about it, but you will not change it. The universe can be described but it is not something you can change, and the unconscious is comparable to that. Laplanche said it's impressive to think that we humans can make our way inside our mind, just like astronomers and astronauts make their way in space, though knowing that we cannot change what is there.

What are we then left with? We are left with the translations—the transductions—that we can achieve, but which are not the unconscious itself. They are *responses* that the translational, transductional psyche can summon in the face of the excitation, of the irritation brought about by the repressed unconscious. The unconscious will always be a provocation requiring that we produce new responses. Of course, we resist that, and we try to maintain a certain stability, even a rigidity against the disturbances brought by the repressed. But, in fact, we are always deported. We are always led astray, adrift by the unconscious. Mind you, this is not all bad; the good news is that this creates the possibility of renewal in our mind during our whole life.

Yet, unfortunately, the clash with the ego can be so strong that the repetition compulsion is elicited and starts working in the opposite direction, because the ego is a structure that struggles to stay as much as possible the same.

The unconscious itself, however, is never fully mated. So, we can come up with new constructions, new scaffoldings around it in response to new events that re-incite us to find meaning. The otherness in the new event resonates with the otherness within us and incites us again to create new symbolizations.

BBT: I'd like to ask you to discuss and elaborate on the difference between the earlier conception of Laplanche's unconscious and the later conception that is found in "Three Meanings of the Term 'Unconscious' in the Framework of the General Theory of Seduction," in *Freud and the Sexual*: One could call it Laplanche's new "structural model" or, as he calls it, "the apparatus of the soul." What are the implications of it? In the paper, he says that using this model allows one to now account for borderline cases and psychotic individuals. Is it safe to say that it's possible in his earlier work that with the model he had of the unconscious, one couldn't account for these two psychopathologies, as it were?

DS: Being someone who, at the very first international meeting around Laplanche's work, in Montréal in 1992, presented a paper about how Laplanche's theory can account for psychosis, I believe that the theory expounded until 1992 already contains what is needed.

BBT: Is this the negation paper?

DS: Yes. The paper entitled '"It was not my mother': from seduction to negation."

When I read Laplanche's paper "Three Meanings of the Term 'Unconscious' in the Framework of the General Theory of Seduction," I was immediately struck by the fact that the diagrams presenting this new topographical model were already familiar to me. I had seen them many years before in Christophe Dejours's work, in a book first published in 1986, *Le corps entre biologie et psychanalyse* [The Body Between Biology and Psychoanalysis], where he presented a very similar model. Dejours worked very closely with Laplanche in the last 15 years or so of Laplanche's life. To me, therefore, this is not an original Laplanchean model. It's Dejours's model imported by Laplanche, although Laplanche mentions that he does not totally agree with Dejours's vocabulary about an "amential unconscious." Laplanche prefers to talk of an *enclaved* unconscious. But this difference in vocabulary is not very important. What matters is if and to what extent this new model is necessary, considering what we already have in Laplanche. Does it really bring something new, or does it represent a kind of reification of the processes that Laplanche has theorized? My view, and this is open for discussion of course, is that there is nothing in the *enclaved* unconscious—or in the new model as a whole—that truly adds to Laplanche's theory.

From an epistemological standpoint, my question is the following: If the "*enclaved* unconscious" is made of memory traces of perceptions that were not at all dealt with by the psyche, that were not subjected to any effort at translation/repression, then how do we know that these recordings even exist? Since they leave no trace whatsoever until they are brought over to the side of translation/repression, how do we know of them? As I said, I don't see what this model adds that is not in the previous theory. To me, the "source objects of the drives," i.e., the untranslatable residues, are just as unfathomable as the elements in the so-called *enclaved* unconscious.

Oddly enough, in the passages where he introduces this notion [Laplanche, 2011, pp. 216–217], Laplanche speaks of the *whole message* as being implanted or intromitted without being translated at all. This is odd because he always insisted that the message he speaks of is but an ordinary message—hence amenable to translation—except for the "parasite" it carries unknowingly. It is therefore strange to posit that there are messages that are stored without being translated at all. When Laplanche gives an example of such messages, he speaks of the "messages of the superego" [p. 218]; this is something he had already addressed in his paper "Implantation, Intromission" and, in my view, the difference does not rest on the nature of the message itself—which can be formally understood yet not amenable to a personal version—but on the "freedom to translate" that we discussed earlier.

I also question the possibility of existence of these totally "raw" *enclaved* elements because, for me, every perception always entails a modicum of translation/transduction—a very primal, rough translation, you would say. As we know, perception is not a passive thing. It is a predictive sampling of the environment; therefore, the child's mind is not a passive receiver of data that could remain *enclaved*. Perception selects and grabs samples of the environment, and therefore also the messages emanating from the adult. Therefore, there's nothing perceived and registered that has not undergone a process of transcription, transduction, translation, *at the stage of perception itself*. To me, it's therefore questionable whether we can speak of something that is somehow registered but exempt of any form of psychic work upon it. We know that something unconscious exists because it somehow manifests itself, and therefore inasmuch as it is subjected to translation/repression.

At this point, you could ask: What about the notion of splitting, of *clivage*, that is involved in that model? Well, *clivage* has been around in Freudian theory since Freud's paper on "Fetishism," as also denial [*Verleugnung*] and rejection [*Verwerfung*, which Lacan translated as "foreclosure"]. These are mechanisms supplemental to translation/repression in the sense that the results of some translations can be so intolerable as to provoke a reaction of denial or rejection. By the way, the phenomenon of denial, which is important in the model we are discussing, supports, I believe, my point in the sense that in order to reject or deny, we must already have a certain, even if a very vague, idea of the unacceptability of what we are perceiving. Therefore, this supposes that, as I was saying, perception itself is always already a form of translation or transduction. This, in my view, runs against the need for a new model. Now, I believe that Dejours, in his 1986 book (re-published in 2018 with a different title), already at the time wanted to introduce a third topographical model in psychoanalysis. There was a kind of race among French analysts to come up with a new model. As for me, I think we have all we need with the first two Freudian models, in Laplanche's work, to account for psychotic and borderline states. I also believe we can invoke splitting, denial, and rejection clinically from within the Translational Model of Laplanche.

To summarize: The thesis of an *enclaved* unconscious, as stated in "Three Meanings of the Term 'Unconscious' in the Framework of the General Theory of Seduction," is to me at the very least worth debating because it appears as contradictory with other Laplanchean tenets.

BBT: I just wanted to clarify or maybe elaborate on one thing. What were the French analysts trying to do with the Third Topographical Model?

DS: Some of them thought a third model was indeed needed to account better for the clinical experience with borderline and psychotic patients. Now, as I said, my contention is that you don't need that. My contention is that, as Lacan has shown, with concepts already present in Freud's writings—such as denial, splitting, and rejection—and with Freud's papers on psychosis, you already have the instruments you need for thinking about the psychotic or the borderline experience. Of course, this requires invoking splitting or rejection as more prevalent than in neurotics—for instance, the splitting of the ego in borderline patients or the rejection of reality in psychosis. But you can do this without the need for a third model.

Laplanche's notion of intromission, which goes back to 1992, is very helpful in understanding the mechanisms of psychosis. The search for a third topology, I think, results, among other things, from a conception of Freud's theory as something layered in a linear progression and a cumulative form of knowledge, like we have in the natural sciences. But I don't think Freudian or Laplanchean theory works that way at all. Freud himself, for instance, in *An Outline of Psychoanalysis*, written near the end of his life, referred to the first and second models, easily shifting from one to the other, using the elements of both models without positing a chasm between them.

BBT: The next question is related to what we were talking about with the *enclaved* unconscious and Dejours's model. Do you think that there are holes or inconsistencies, incongruencies in Laplanche's work? Aside from that one that you just discussed?

DS: There probably are, but I haven't looked for them actively. It would be preposterous, I think, to assert that Laplanche can be totally free of contradictions. The one that immediately comes to mind is the question whether implantation—and this was brought to my attention by Avgi Saketopoulou—involves itself a certain violence, which is not readily obvious in the theory. Mind you, Laplanche clearly speaks of implantation as a trauma, a generic trauma, but he does not insist on the violent aspect of implantation.

This could be one possible question, but it is a rather minor point. I am sure that if we looked at Laplanche's work from up close in the way he looked at Freud's work from up close—and by the way, Laplanche himself asked of us that we put him back to work, that we identify the points in his theory that need re-elaboration, that need revisiting, and so on—I am sure that we can find problematic elements. I, for one, have spoken earlier of "transduction" as more appropriate than "translation." This could probably be the starting point of a wider discussion.

BBT: Perhaps we can discuss applying Laplanche's theory to the clinical vignettes or using the clinical vignettes in any way, shape, or form. You have mentioned how it shows the biases of the clinician, but there is a theoretical position that I believe you take on this issue.

DS: I believe that we must ask ourselves what are the vignettes destined to do? When we do group clinical discussions and the like, and perhaps this is also your experience, we easily fall in the trap of putting ourselves in the analyst's position and start to think or say, "In your place, I would've said this or that," or "I think that your patient was saying this or that to you." Forgetting, that is, that we were not the target of the patient's transference, that we have an outsider's look at the material, and that we were not concerned and not pressured by the patient's transferential movements. Laplanche was extremely critical of this. It's never a matter of "Here is what I would have said, or here is what you should hear in what your patient said."

We are allowed to speculate, of course, and to imagine, but I think that we must always be aware that we are then responding with our own transference to the analyst that is presenting the case and not addressing the case itself as if we had truly been in the analyst's armchair. It follows that, in terms of the validity of the clinical example offered to the discussion, we are dealing with a continuing process of triggering things in us that are not necessarily linked with the case material.

Many years ago, when I was the editor of a section in *The International Journal of Psychoanalysis* called "The Analyst at Work," we had a discussion about what a clinical paper needs in order to be useful and interesting. I then used the metaphor of "live wires," that is, the paper, the recounting of the clinical case, must still contain some live wires. This was another word for untranslated elements in the material reported, for things that seem to be calling for our attention, that seem to provoke in us something that we don't readily understand, but which invite us to try and elaborate more, knowing that we are the ones transferring on the paper. Again, we are not the targets of the transference by the patient that is talked about in the paper. This creates a wholly new situation, which has only indirect links with the original case.

It's a question of the locus of experience, of what experience we are talking about. If I try to justify or even to illustrate my theory with a clinical case, I will miss the point in the sense that my clinical vignette will arouse in the reader a new set of responses and will provoke their own theory, and therefore this starts a kind of infinite digression, I would say, from one theory to the other. Like it or not, we each have a certain theory, whether explicit or implicit. Better to have a clear theory than only an implicit one, but we always have a theory. Because of this, it's an impossible task, in our field, to try and clinically prove or even illustrate a specific theory because our case material will always be addressed by each analyst in the audience from their own theoretical standpoint.

Whereas I think that a good metapsychological paper, without any reference to a specific case, will by itself speak to the analyst's personal experience. If the paper addresses an actual problem, an actual issue in a rigorous and useful way, it will summon in the reader's mind clinical situations that speak to them. This, at least, was my experience with the most important authors that I met: Laplanche, Aulagnier, or even Winnicott. Even today, when I read them, their theoretical formulations resonate with this or that experience that I had with my own patients. But even so, what I get in the end is my own version of their theory. This is a reminder that we do not have in our field what they have in physics, that is, the crucial experiment or the equation that really fixates the matter on paper, such as $E=mc^2$. We don't have that in psychoanalysis because we are not dealing with material that can be calculated.

BBT: Related to what you're bringing up is the question of research in psychoanalysis. You brought up a good metapsychological paper. Does it need a clinical case? How would you describe or think about an effective Laplanchean style and method of going about research in psychoanalysis? How is that different from other disciplines and psychoanalytic research in general?

DS: I think you are addressing one of Laplanche's major contributions, the one expounded in the already-mentioned paper, "Interpreting (with) Freud." It's a paper that I call "programmatic" in the sense that it contains Laplanche's research program. There, he explains what it is to use Freud's theoretical apparatus—the methodological apparatus that Freud bequeathed us—and to turn it *toward,* and if need be, *against* Freud himself. This to me is Laplanche's major lesson, the most important of the three great things that he brought—the two others being the Translational Model of the mind and the General Theory of Seduction.

As already said, Laplanche's method can be applied in rereading Laplanche himself, or Winnicott, or whoever. I used it, for instance, with Winnicott's paper "The Use of an Object." Laplanche says, whenever you detect textual or theoretical events, oddities, contradictions, second thoughts, etc., stop, think, and dig deeper in that area, because a good author does not create these incidents without a reason. Therefore, we are asked to re-examine the whole context. If need be, we will be called upon to reformulate things by unearthing issues, problems that were not apparent at first sight. It's really a method that starts from small indexes, small hints that something more lurks underneath. This, I think, is the way that we can do what is called "conceptual research" in psychoanalysis and which is using metapsychology about metapsychology itself. It's a unique case of continuous self-reflection and self-investigation of psychoanalysis.

BBT: I'm going to make a fairly big pivot and ask a different sort of question. In what way does stressing the sadomasochistic dimension of the unconscious allow for a movement away from normative family structures and gender issues in sexuality, reproduction, and love in the common sense?

DS: There are at least two questions in your question. One of them is about stressing the sadomasochistic dimension. Yes, you could say that Laplanche does that. I personally think that it goes beyond the sadomasochistic dimension. Recently, I have been working on the idea that if the sexual drive is what egregiously disturbs the subject, it's not because of its being "sexual" in the trivial sense, but because the sexual drive is enrolled into the structure of power, into the search for power over another subject, reducing that other subject to the state of an object, and what is more, of a part-object. The sadomasochistic dimension is but one manifestation of that. But the exertion of power can manifest itself in other manners as well. To go back to your previous question, here is another debate that could be opened: whether all violence is necessarily sadomasochistic. Laplanche, I think, would say yes. Laurence Kahn is another major author who thinks, for instance, that Nazism was not specifically a sadomasochistic enterprise, that there was a kind of "cold violence" unaccountable for in sexual terms (see her book *What Nazism Did to Psychoanalysis*, which recently came out in English).

I believe that the drive which concerns us most is the one that Laplanche called the *sexual* death drive. I recently called it a *sexual drive for power*, not for the sake of introducing a new drive. Not at all. It's the same drive we are talking about—a drive that does not comply with the quest for stability on the part of the ego. It's the drive that disturbs and constantly provokes new responses; its source is the repressed.

Laplanche has reminded us that when we speak of the drive, or the repressed, or the unconscious, we do this from the point of view of the ego. It's always the ego speaking, because what we know of a drive is that it disturbs the ego. (This, by the way, could be another argument against the *enclaved* unconscious model: an unconscious with no drive?) Therefore, what we know most is the disturbance experienced by the ego, so that when the drive meets the ego, so to speak, it's not a pure drive we experience. It is always intermixed with the ego's efforts at mastering it. The best way the ego finds in trying to master the drive is by mastering the object, the outer object, by trying to create a situation where narcissistic omnipotence is at work. A third concept, however, must be invoked: *Bemächtigungstrieb*, that is, in Strachey's translation, the "drive for mastery," but whose more accurate translation is the "drive for power" (*Macht*). Then, with the convergence of these three aspects (the *Sexual*, narcissistic omnipotence, and *Bemächtigungstrieb*), you obtain a *sexual drive for power,* which is the *sexual* death drive under another name, but made more explicit in terms of what is so disturbing about it.

As for the life drives, taken in themselves, as analysts we're not as concerned with them. (This is not as simple as I appear to say and would require a long digression.) What is specific to us humans are the sexual drives—Laplanche's *Sexual*, with a capital S—i.e., not what pertains to *sexuality*, but as the *disturbance*, the turmoil, which, by the way, can disturb sexuality itself. As for the sadomasochistic dimension, as I said, I do wonder if this says the whole story about the *sexual* death drive, but it is certainly one of its major manifestations.

How does it allow for a movement away from normative family structures? The *sexual* drive has from the get-go allowed for such a deviance; that is noticeable already in Freud's *Three Essays on the Theory of Sexuality*. Even if in the third essay, as Laplanche has shown, Freud falls back on normativity—the two first essays amply show how the *Sexual* in humans is always already deviant.

What we have then is a disturbing element within us which forces us to find ways of containing it, of dealing with it, of surviving its disorganizing effects and keeping together something that pertains to the interests of the ego. Now, when this is attempted, a new field of struggle is opened where the question is: What structures do we need for that purpose? In whose interest are these structures brought about? In the history of humankind, a main current has been, and still is, the patriarchal current. (It seems dubious that there were matriarchal societies.) Whatever the case, we have a patriarchal response to the problem of the drive, a structure that has been operating for millennia. But it so happens that in the last decades or centuries, two or three centuries at most, the reflection, the discoveries, and the critical look at these traditional responses about how to contain the potential destructive effect of the drive, have given way to new models, new ideas.

I wouldn't say that it's stressing the sadomasochistic dimension per se that did this. The *sexual* death drive, the sadomasochistic dimension, the *sexual drive for power* have always been around. The question is: Are our ways of dealing with it happening today in a context such that we can now opt for other models? Moving away from the traditional family structures, I think, is more due to the new tools that we have at our disposal, intellectual tools, but also political and technical tools.

BBT: How do Laplanche's General Theory of Seduction and the Translational Model of Repression offer a different perspective to the clinical vignettes? Considering this difference, how would you compare Laplanche to classical and contemporary Freudian theory, Kleinian theory, Bionian theory, self-psychology, intersubjectivity, etc.?

DS: I think that the most important thing is to become aware of the seductive effect. We discussed previously the seductive effect of the analyst's installing of the analytic frame, the analytic "tub." The way in which the analyst, by creating this tub, invites a reopening of the Fundamental Anthropological Situation, as Laplanche called it. Therefore, this changes to a certain extent the analyst's stance regarding transference, as Laplanche has illustrated in his imaginary dialogue at the beginning of his paper "Transference: Its Provocation by the Analyst," in *The Unfinished Copernican Revolution*. A good example of radical de-centeredness.

The analyst says: "You are taking me for someone else"—this is the classical analyst speaking—"I am not the person you think I am." And the analysand responds: "Exactly—the other in the originary relation was not the person I thought, so I'm perfectly right to take you for someone else" [Laplanche & Thurston, 2020, p. 515]. Here you have, I think, one of the important outlooks on de-centeredness. We are always other; from the very start, the primal other is not the person the child, or himself, thinks it is. The analyst too is not what he thinks, but that's not a problem. That's the real situation. We are not in contact with the person we think we are dealing with because the otherness is always moving us astray from what we consider as being the facts, the reality of the situation.

Now, this may sound very abstract, but think of the attitude of the analyst regarding a transferential feeling. Here again is another topic about which I used clinical material: the case of a delusional transference, namely erotomania. A patient, very early on, started to be firmly convinced that I had taken her into treatment because the moment I saw her, I fell in love with her. I struggled with that transference, with her insistence on it, for several years. I tried, not overtly of course, to get around that by interpreting, for instance:

"You believe this because you need me to be the mother that was not available to you," and so on. But nothing worked until I asked myself, in the wake of Freud's idea, *What if this patient is in some way right?* Not that I am in love with her; not that I took her in treatment because I was in love with her; but what if what Freud says in "Mourning and Melancholia," that *in some way* the patient must be right, also applies to the present delusions?

This totally changed the game. I don't know exactly what changed in me that was felt by her, but she became much less harassing toward me. She stopped trying to make me confess that I was in love with her. We started doing more useful work, probably because my personal attitude toward her, or toward what I called her delusional transference, was not to consider it delusional anymore, but to tacitly give her credit that "in some way" she was right in transforming me into someone who was in love with her. This, in a very minute and difficult-to-pinpoint manner, brought us smoothly to termination.

I had the opportunity to see this patient twice after the end of her therapy and to see that she was faring well. She was much warmer in her relationship and more effective in dealing with things that could have been difficult for her to manage before. What I'm saying here is that the way you work with your patients changes when you come to realize that they are somehow right in taking you for someone else. It's a matter, therefore, of taking responsibility in a certain way for what we have provoked in them in the transference. This, I think, is a possible example of what Laplanche's theory may change in terms of practice.

Bibliography

Aulagnier, P. (2001). *The violence of interpretation: From pictogram to statement*. Brunner-Routledge.

Dejours, C., & Dagognet, F. (1986). *Le corps entre biologie et psychanalyse: Essai d'interprétation comparée*. Payot.

Freud, S. (1927). Fetishism. In J. Strachey (Ed. & Trans.), *The standard edition of the complete psychological works of Sigmund Freud* (Vol. 21, pp. 147–157). Hogarth Press and the Institute of Psycho-Analysis.

Freud, S. (1953). Mourning and melancholia. In J. Strachey (Ed. & Trans.), SE (Vol. 14, pp. 243–258). Hogarth Press.

Freud, S. (2016). *Three essays on the theory of sexuality: The 1905 edition* (U. Kistner, Trans.). Verso.

Freud, S., & Ragg-Kirkby, H. (2003). *An outline of psychoanalysis*. Penguin.

Kahn, L., & Weller, A. (2023). *What Nazism did to psychoanalysis*. Routledge, Taylor & Francis Group.

Laplanche, J. (2011). Psychoanalysis and psychotherapy. Edited by John Fletcher. In *Freud and the sexual: Essays, 2000–2006* (pp. 344–351). The Unconscious in Translation.

Laplanche, J. (2020). Intromission and implantation (L. Thurston, Trans.). In J. Laplanche & L. Thurston, *The unfinished Copernican revolution: Selected works, 1967–1992* (pp. 73–88). The Unconscious in Translation.

Laplanche, J., & House, J. (2016). *New foundations for psychoanalysis*. The Unconscious in Translation.

Laplanche, J., & Mehlman, J. (2015). *Between seduction and inspiration: Man*. The Unconscious in Translation.

Laplanche, J., & Thurston, L. (2020). *The unfinished Copernican revolution: Selected works, 1967–1992*. The Unconscious in Translation.

Lyotard, J.-F. (2007). *The differend: Phrases in dispute*. University of Minnesota Press.

Scarfone, D. (2002). "It was not my mother": From seduction to negation. *New Formations, 48*, 69–76.

Winnicott, D. W. (1969). The use of an object. *The International Journal of Psychoanalysis, 50*(4), 711–716.

5 Luiz Carlos Tarelho

São Paulo, Brazil

Interview conducted in Portuguese and translated into English.

Bryan Batista-Thomas: You had wanted to start with the following questions: (1) How does the reality of the message, and the materiality of it, cause Laplanche's theory to be one that is nonsubjective? (2) Given that Laplanche did not study newborns, and his theory is not one of developmental psychology, how does his theory necessitate and work with historical foundations—considering both the clinical context of the analysand and within culture? and (3) For you, what is an effective, and Laplanchean *style* of going about research in psychoanalysis? How is this different from other disciplines and psychoanalytic research in general?

Luiz Carlos Tarelho: I took the liberty of calling them fundamentals in order to organize myself. I would say that an important aspect to consider is Laplanche's philosophical background. He was, in the beginning at least, in the '60s, '70s, called a philosopher psychoanalyst in France, an expression that wasn't always positive. It had a tone that was a little bit judgmental, debauched. But he didn't mind because, for him, it was correct.

In the beginning, he has a few lines in *The Unfinished Copernican Revolution*, where he says, "It is like this relationship between theory and practice has a philosophical dimension." He positions himself from there. But it is also important to remember that he left philosophy and his philosophical training with the firm purpose of being able to contribute to renewing and deepening knowledge about the human being. Laplanche wanted to leave behind a legacy. But it is interesting how paradoxical it is that it was not in philosophy

DOI: 10.4324/9781032670287-6

that he saw this possibility. We can't forget that he was a student of Maurice Merleau-Ponty.

BBT: Right.

LCT: Merleau-Ponty was a philosopher that had interlocutors both in psychology and psychoanalysis. Within that philosophical training that Laplanche had, there was a very strong influence of Merleau-Ponty. Why psychoanalysis? Why not philosophy?

Psychoanalysis came to reveal the existence of a hitherto unknown domain of reality connected to the unconscious, which Freud called psychic reality—a reality as hard as iron. As he says, different from external, material reality, but also different from psychological reality, a reality marked by meaning. An egoic reality, the reality of consciousness. Laplanche says how Freud is going to get lost. This third dimension of reality is where I think Laplanche comes in to contribute. The knowledge of such a reality is new—something that is in the psyche, maybe even in the foundation of the psyche. But it functions as a thing, as a causality that is not in external reality, nor in science. This idea of causality was abandoned by science, but it remains pertinent to our discussion about this third level of reality. That is, of something that is in the foundation of the psyche—that belongs to the order of the psyche but is not mediated by meaning. It comes from the world of communication but has lost the ability to communicate.

What exactly am I calling a foundation then? Foundation is from the author's point of view, their trajectory. As a philosopher, Laplanche discovers psychoanalysis. He will work on psychoanalytic thinking about this contribution that psychoanalysis brought, which is the discovery of this new domain of reality—from the epistemological point of view, to sustain the scientificity of this discipline, which is the other great challenge. I think that these two challenges, parallel paths, are two central axes of his thought. A novelty, this domain of reality, this level of reality, and at the same time, the need to show that this discipline has the right to occupy a space in the scientific world. From there, he goes inside psychoanalysis, not outside. The first part of *New Foundations for Psychoanalysis*, "Catharsis," is to show the external foundations, that is, biology, genetics, linguistics from Lacan, the mechanism that Freud also used from a physics perspective, etc.

Psychoanalysis, if it is to search outside of these domains that are connected, loses its essence. The first part of the book shows that it makes no sense to search in the connected domains for the foundation. Laplanche was asked, "Does searching from within mean searching in one's own practice?" Laplanche responded that this was Freud's claim at some point. However, Laplanche points out that a practice that would base its object on the practice itself is somewhat redundant. Practice is important, but for Laplanche, the foundation must be somewhere else. The foundation must be in the human being itself. That's the direction he is heading. If psychoanalysis discovered something new, unheard of about the human being, it is in this humanity itself.

The analytic method, given this interrelation, is directly linked to the object. The method is the road to know the object. It reveals the nature, the specificity of this object, which is the unconscious. That is, its belonging to another level of reality, which intervenes not through meaning, but through force. Through causality, as Laplanche says, the drive. With that reasoning, Laplanche would say the intention is to show that psychoanalysis has its foundation in that very domain of reality, which is the unconscious, the message, the signifier of that meaning whose origin needs to be explained.

BBT: Needing or not needing explanation?

LCT: Needing the origin to be explained. The function of theory, or one of the functions, is to explain how it constitutes this reality, this object. Also, the method. Why do I need this specific method to yield to this reality, to access it? It is in this explanation that we find the possibility for psychoanalysis to affirm itself as an independent consciousness, even as a science and as an independent science, independent of the related domains of biology, of language, etc. This is where one of your questions comes in—"Given that Laplanche did not study newborns, and his theory is not one of developmental psychology, how does his theory necessitate and work with historical foundations?"

Laplanche didn't work with children. He is not going to settle for taking psychology as a foundation, because it's another reality. Therefore, what is the need for the historical foundations of his issue? He explains this in a paper called "Levels of Proof."

BBT: "Levels of Proof" is in *Freud and the* Sexual.

LCT: He will say that it is necessary to do psychoanalytic research on children. That is why he admired Silvia Bleichmar's work so much. She was a child analyst and was thinking about this theory of the constitution of the unconscious in a way that was very close to Laplanche's. She would diverge in some points, but she was an example to him of how to do science. But there it is science; it is not research—a research in the scientific model. It is research based on clinical practice. In Laplanche's mind, I think that this was one of the sources of research, clinical practice. But he could also do research in the classical sense of the term. This form of research goes through the method. To yield to this reality, there is no other method. To do research in psychoanalysis implies following the criteria of science. Laplanche would say his great interlocutor was Karl Popper. For him, psychoanalysis needs to follow the criteria of falsification, of testing; otherwise, it's not science.

BBT: Right.

LCT: It needs to follow the classic criteria of a science. But it will need the analytic method. It will have to insert in this process an analytic method, that is, a listening that can perceive this unconscious, or this object that is not of the order of meaning. It is not of the order of physical matter. It is not of the order of the biological, communicative language, of meaning, or generator of meaning. This level of reality is transversal to psychological reality and material reality. Transversal in that it circulates on these two levels, so it's just the analytic method. You must add the analytic method to the classical scientific method to be able to do research. The clinical is a way to do research because there you have at least one of the basic conditions, which is the analytic method. Of course, you don't have the other criteria, let's say the issue of controls. You have a little bit of control because this is in a session. Theoretically, it is based on a constancy of factors. Within the epistemological perspective, there is first the need to show that psychoanalysis is a science. Because it works with real, concrete objects. It has this concern that we cannot accept that because it is not directly observable, we must appeal to something that belongs to the order of the mythical.

There is a current in psychoanalysis that goes that way. We cannot observe it directly, why? Because of the idea that it is a reconstruction. Therefore, you don't have access to it. You can only imagine what it is. Laplanche was against this view and said that's a means to deny that there is a concrete object. That concrete object is not of the order of meaning as hermeneutics wants. As the Lacanians want. That is where the great divergence with Lacan began. There is no chain of meaning in the unconscious for Laplanche. Or a second chain, or the greater chain, if we think in Lacanian terms—the chain that founded all the others. For Laplanche, it is the real concrete, but it is not of the order of meaning. Because repression operated, causing a dislocation, a kind of transmutation.

It takes something that is of the order of the psyche and transforms it into something that belongs to the order of things. The signifier no longer has the capacity to signify. Then it is sort of removed from the context, from this symbolizing context. It becomes something like any other and operates according to the principle of causality. That is the dislocation. This is the purpose of theory. Theory is a model, as Laplanche says, "in the Popperian sense." Every model is hypothetical. It must be susceptible to falsification.

BBT: I'd like to come back to some things. You were talking a little bit about Popper's methodology of falsification, about the third reality, and the aspects necessary to do research. Laplanche said that you need to add the analytic method, and one of the places where you could do this is in the clinical realm. Where would be another place, another way? Another question about Silvia Bleichmar: how did she do research with children in this method?

LCT: Let's start with Bleichmar. She didn't do research in the classical sense of scientific research. She built everything from the clinical. There you're using exclusively the analytic method. Laplanche didn't go as far as describing, "Well, research has to be done like this." He said, "There has to be research in psychoanalysis too." As psychologists do, as other domains of science do, and psychoanalysis is one. If it is a domain of science, it also needs to do research. When he talks, he thinks a lot about observation.

I think it needs to be an observation, maybe longitudinal, and this is the advantage of clinical practice, because you accompany a child over a relatively medium time span. Laplanche didn't describe it, but we can imagine that, besides clinical research, it is necessary to do classical research by observing children, with an emphasis on the specific object of psychoanalysis which will be constituted, the unconscious.

BBT: Understood.

LCT: How is repression going to be produced? Going further, repression is not directly observable.

BBT: Exactly.

LCT: Even if you observe a child full time, you're not going to see repression occurring. We're going to see changes in behavior, the construction of the child's theories, the models that he uses to explain his own life. Then the analytic method is necessary, because, when you are faced with the construction, the model built by the child, you must deconstruct it to understand what is behind it, what led to it. On the other hand, we must imagine what kind of message we addressed to the child. This is the great difference of a Laplanchean clinical approach. It is the capacity of the analyst and the patient to retrieve the context in which he constituted himself, including the messages that he received.

I would say what characterizes a Laplanchean analysis is the possibility of being able to retrieve something that comes from the other, in the form of a message, of an injunction, of an exigency. I refer to section six in *New Foundations for Psychoanalysis*, which is called "Foundations and Historical Origin: Psychoanalysis and Psychology," located in "Catharsis." What are the fundamentals for Laplanche? He says that there are two basic historical foundations, one is the appearance of the psychoanalytic subject with the unconscious. But this appearance of the psychoanalytic subject of the unconscious, of repression, is inserted into another, broader history, which is the history of the individual, of the child. It includes a history of the psychological, developmental psychology, and self-preservative, or attachment. It has two foundations that are mixed up: the developmental psychological foundation and the foundation of the creation of the unconscious. They are two different levels of reality. This is why he says, "Well, clinical practice alone cannot be the foundation. Because practice also goes back to the past." As we have just said with the example here, this practice, this analysis can only be understood in light of what happened there in childhood, and in childhood you have a process of genetic development and, along with it, seduction.

You have a genesis, the history in the genetic sense. In the sense of the constitution. From the psychological side, it is inscribed in the biological genetic process, in part at least. You have a certain process that will progress, with some interaction with the social world. In the case of the psychology of the unconscious, for Laplanche there is no such genesis in the biological sense; it is not inscribed in a program. It is a process that, although it is concrete and factual, is not directly observable. Therefore, repression is a factual thing; it is something that happened.

It also does not happen at a specific point. It is a process, just as the constitution of the "I" occurs in a process. But it is necessary to reconstitute the context. Because it is the context that establishes and confers specificity to this object, to this genesis. This specific historical time Laplanche will call "originary." The idea of originary is important; it is very well described in this chapter of *New Foundations for Psychoanalysis*. He will even say, "The originary is a deepening of the notion of reality." It is linked to time, to fact, to an event, but he deepens it. For him, psychoanalysis is concerned with this originary. This is important, so that it is the constitution of the unconscious of sexuality and together with this history. These two historical foundations, the psychological and the psychoanalytic, he says, are two foundations—one of the self-preservatives and one of sexuality. These two foundations together constitute a phenomenological finding. It is a fundamental phenomenological finding that is the condition of helplessness of the human being when he comes into the world. His complete dependence on adults. Later, he will call this the Fundamental Anthropological Situation.

The notion of passivity for him is essential. It's not about phenomenological passivity, that is, about acting; that's not the essence of passivity. He will turn to philosophy to talk about the adult's knowing more and the child's not knowing. Passivity is this absolute inadequacy to deal with the sexual. Because from the point of view of attachment, Laplanche says, "You can't say that the child is totally passive." He will appeal there. He says, "You have to turn to research," developmental psychology, attachment theory. There's been research showing that the child seems active, reacts, interacts, and communicates, and that's why he's going to say something along the lines of José Carlos Calich's work; it translates too. That is, there's something instinctive in these instinctive assemblies, in this self-preservative plane, before the constitution of the instanced self. That is, the topographical division, there is something originating in the child that enables it to symbolize. For the child, the question is not that it has to open itself to the world. The big problem is to close itself because it comes open to the world. The question is the constitution of an internal space that needs a closure. So much so that Laplanche plays with the expression of Winnicott. He says that the big problem is not the constitution of a "not-me possession," but the opposite—of a space of a "me possession." A space of my own. This passivity at this originary level, alongside the inevitable activity of the adult with his unconscious, that's when you think, the child is passive because he doesn't have an unconscious. The adult is active, not only because he acts but also because he has an unconscious—it's the meeting of these two realities. This unconscious that infiltrates into this relationship, without the adult's knowledge, constitutes the essence of the seductive fact. For Laplanche, this is the great engine of seduction that he will call "enigma." There is a whole issue up here—many people don't like the term.

BBT: "Enigma"?

LCT: Of the term "enigma," yes.

BBT: Why not?

LCT: Because "enigma" gets too stuck in this world of meaning, in the world of the known, in a way.

BBT: Then the preference would be "message"?

LCT: No. That is why Laplanche will say neither the signifier nor the message is enigmatic. I think that the important thing is that the motor of the symbolizing translational process is that it is deposited in the child that already operates as a strange object. It produces an unbalance. This is fundamental for him. This enigma comes to disturb the relative balance that exists on the level of the self-preservative, which tends to fix homeostasis, and that will require a work of contention. Although we can say, at the beginning, that it is more by way of the body that this contention will be produced. As much as autoeroticism is a translation that is fundamentally corporal, and Laplanche is open to this, he speaks about how both messages come first in a nonsymbolic or nonlinguistic way. It is a corporal message. It is a body-to-body translation that takes place between the adult and the child before anything else.

The enigma is based on an interpellation without content. Because the enigma is basically this—it is an interpellation that comes along with the message, but what interpellates is not the message, it is the signifier. It is that which says nothing; it only interpellates, so this is what is going to drive the process of symbolization and is going to transform itself. Laplanche uses this expression as a fixed motor, that is, the base, which is the foundation of the seduction, and what will also become the source of the drive.

My proposal is that we now develop what I would call a second block: concerning the clinic, the method, the technique, which for me is a continuation of the previous block on foundations. Remembering that Laplanche insists a lot on this, and that Freud, when he goes on to define psychoanalysis, starts with the method. Theory must be able to explain this joint necessity of the object and the method. We can say, "It's the singularity of the object—the singularity that is the unconscious that justifies the specificity of the method." A singularity that comes from the process of constitution of this object, which is repression. It makes and produces all this transformation. Laplanche even calls it displacement, which causes the signifier to cease to be a signifier. This signifier ceases to belong to the communicative world, to the extent that a loss of reference is produced. Then it will also imply an absence of meaning and of associative chains in this universe, in this other level of reality.

Freud discovers this level of reality, invents a method to have access to it, but then he introduces the complexes. He is going to need another method that is hermeneutic. Laplanche points out how Freud realizes this contradiction; he may not have been an epistemologist, but he knew what he was talking about. Freud realized that there was a contradiction between the two methods. He made a choice favoring the hermeneutic method as compared to the analytic method. Laplanche puts the analytic method at the origin. Because he is going to invert it, so it is the repressed unconscious that is at the origin. It is not the complexes that are at the core of the unconscious. It is the repressed: the signifier of this signified, it is the absence of meaning.

There in the beginning, when Freud was building the metapsychology, he was faced with this absence of meaning, which is what demanded the creation of a specific method and it is associative of the associative. By means of free association, he aims to retrieve not a concealed, latent meaning, but fragments that were excluded from a signifying plot and that can only be accessed through associations with conscious or preconscious elements. This is what explains the analytic method invented by Freud. Because this third domain of reality formed by signifiers has lost its relationship with the world of the senses, of signification, and they now act as a thing. Laplanche puts the repressed at the origin of the drive, and the analytic method as the true psychoanalytic method. He will put the translational theory at the center, allowing us to resituate the mytho-symbolic as a connecting element.

BBT: Can you say more about how the mytho-symbolic serves the function as the link for the translational theory?

LCT: It is the translational theory that allows us to resituate this whole mytho-symbolic universe. Laplanche is going to make the following displacement: all the myths, Oedipus, for example, these translational models, are connecting elements instead of the foundation of the unconscious. Of course, Freud discovered something important with Oedipus. Laplanche is not questioning the existence of Oedipus. He is questioning the place given to Oedipus by Freud throughout post-Freudian psychoanalysis—the place of a foundation.

Laplanche says Oedipus has a function. But it is a function of connection. It cannot be the core of the unconscious. It is not the source of the drive. It serves to connect. Where to situate Oedipus? Where to situate the mytho-symbolic? It's not on the side of the repressed. It's on the side of the repressor, of that which represses.

Going back to the idea of realism, because we started off with that, scientism has to do with realism, but this realism is based on three axes. The first axis is the genesis, which is identifiable by observing the unconscious, the drive, even if indirectly. Laplanche says, "Well, of course we won't be able to reconstruct point 'x' where repression happened, but we can reconstruct the process indirectly." What he calls historical. The second axis has a materiality. It is not a myth; it is based on a concrete element, and it is the signifier of that signified. Moreover, it is a materiality that helps to explain the functioning of the unconscious, of the drive. The third axis of this realism is in the method. The question of the method, the technique of the clinic. It is a method capable of accessing this material. A method that also needs to be explained. This method cannot be based on guesswork. It is not by intuition; it's a concrete method.

Why is the method scientific? First, it can be reproduced—so you see that Laplanche has a Popperian inspiration. That's what the analytical method is—it is not for a specific thing; anyone can do this experiment anywhere in the world. Second, it has a neutrality, because the method itself cannot interfere in the object. It cannot pre-determine the object like hermeneutics does. Hermeneutics brings an interpretative code. The analytical method does not bring a key. On the contrary, it will allow us to find something individual and specific to each subject, and it succeeds in doing this. It is effective in what it aims to do. It allows us to access this material without pre-determining, predicting this material.

Now, the word "interpret" is sometimes misunderstood and misused by the analyst. Interpreting fits very well into hermeneutic work. Hermeneutics is also an interpretation. It is an interpretation with a pre-established key; the analytical interpretation is without a key. Laplanche uses a metaphor and says, "If we could compare hermeneutics with a key to open a lock." He says, "This is the big problem of hermeneutics; the same key that can be used to open a lock is also used to close it, lock it."

The analytic interpretation, in this metaphor, needs to function like a screwdriver; it's going to disassemble the lock, that is, without a code. It disassembles the lock in order to allow everything to pass through, and not only that which that key would allow one to see. To interpret in the Freudian analytical sense, is very specific: It's to decompose, to analyze. In psychoanalysis, we are decomposing the egoic syntheses, the connections, especially the symptomatic ones that led the subject to seek analysis.

BBT: What would an analytical interpretation look like as compared to a hermeneutic interpretation?

LCT: The example that comes to my mind, is never to say, in the matter of transference, "You are treating me as your mother." For him, this is a

> hermeneutic interpretation. We are opening, but closing at the same time, saying that at the origin of the transference, there is the relationship with the mother, and the patient is just transferring the figure. This is kind of obvious, it's what he will call the filled-in transference. The big question is, why is the transference taking place? This is the hollowed-out transference, open, in the void. Why is the analysand led to take the figure of the analyst as their mother? A screwdriver is needed to dismantle this lock, the key to the lock wanted. Instead of saying, "You are treating me as your mother," an analytic interpretation would be, "Why are you taking me as your mother?" Rather than giving an answer, you posed another question to go beyond.

The analyst has three basic functions: First, to be the pilot of the method. He is the one who needs to know the moment to cut, to deconstruct, and to point out a synthesis that needs to be undone. It's not that we cannot talk about Oedipus, but the analyst needs to show, "Look you are producing a synthesis here, an Oedipal reproduction. We need to understand why. Let's take it apart to see."

Second, the analyst also needs to be the guarantor of containment, to preserve the analytic space, *le baquet* [the tub]. It's not possible to talk, delivering that disconnecting work which is analysis, if there is not a space that is going to guarantee that the subject continues. I mean that the person is not going to unravel, they are not going to disintegrate. Analysis is always a game of balance between these two movements: *sexual* life drive and the *sexual* death drive—connection and disconnection. That's why the analyst is the pilot; he must know when to accelerate, brake, poke the wound. When he must comfort. Laplanche brings back Winnicott here, and the notion of holding is fundamental. Without that, you can't do analysis, and it's one of the criticisms that he makes to Lacanism. One of the things that Lacanism lacks the most is holding. Holding is a series of elements that are going to constitute security.

Third, the analyst also must be the guardian of enigma, and there, at a certain point in one of your questions, you raise the issue of Laplanchean ethics. I would say the foundation of Laplanchean ethics is there: the analyst as the guardian of enigma. Why is that? Because that is what guarantees transference. That is what moves the individual, moves the subject. It is the relation to enigma, which is the motor of the drive, of transference. Specifically, the motor of the hollowed-out transference, which is the real motor of transference. There is only filled-in transference, there is only Oedipus, because you have the hollowed-out transference, because you have enigma. Respecting enigma, he says, is respecting the other in me. Look at this ethical question: I will only be able to respect the other, and the other of the other, if I respect the other in me. Put another way, my tolerance to difference passes through the recognition of enigma. Passes through the recognition of otherness, that otherness is constitutive. It is in all of us. Because alterity is a motor, it does not have to be fought.

Lacan says it is our dependence on the meaning of the world, on the symbolism, that is the real castration. That is why it is structural. It isn't specific to an individual; it belongs to everyone, to the human being. Laplanche didn't develop it, but I'm trying to put this into his mouth—he would say this: Refusal is the question of otherness. Therefore, this *enclave* needs to be thought of as a refusal. This is a refusal of otherness in me, that is, I must deny this otherness all the time. We all need it, and that is narcissism. That is the self, the ideals; they are constituted to deny this otherness. When this works on the narcissistic level, things work well. The big question is when the person cannot handle this refusal of this narcissistic form.

Laplanche will say, "This can happen in other places." The analytic situation is not an exclusive place of transference for the reopening of the original situation. For example, it is reopened in relation with the cultural; it is a privileged place of transference, because the cultural embodies this unknown other all the time. What is the difference between analysis and the analytic space? It's the analysis, the differential of the analytic space. That is why the analyst is the pilot of the method. Because without analysis, there is no process of deconstruction, or at least there is not a technically assisted deconstruction with a therapeutic goal, in the sense of healing. He says, "Analysis is dangerous." Because it's the work of the *sexual* death drive, and this work of the *sexual* death drive, out of the context of the analytical situation, generally leads to confusion and a certain complete ambivalence everywhere, since there is no containment. When you open yourself to someone, and that someone allows you to put your finger on the wound, it usually doesn't end well. In the analytic space, it's part of this space, and it needs to be understood because it is not self-evident. It's something that is part of the explanation of how the process works.

BBT: Let's speak a little about sadomasochism, and if you could answer the following questions: (1) How does Laplanche's Translational Model of Repression represent a refusal of a psyche/body dichotomy? How does this refusal permeate through his work, like in the case of a radical failure of translation? (2) Related to the previous question, in the refusal of the internal and external, where for Laplanche the external other becomes the internal other, what are the implications for clinical practice? For example, how does the analyst understand the session and/or the analysand's material? (3) How do the issues of gender, power, race, and class come up in your cultural context as it relates to Laplanche's theory? In what ways does Laplanche's theory address these issues? (4) For you, what is an effective, and Laplanchean, *style* of going about research in psychoanalysis? How is this different from other disciplines and psychoanalytic research in general?

LCT: I think this is one of the most interesting questions that you put there in your conceptualizations. Perhaps it is a little risky to think about the masochistic dimension of the unconscious, of sexuality. More of

> sexuality than of the unconscious. I would emphasize the masochistic dimension of the unconscious and of sexuality in its origin. I think this is what Laplanche considers the first manifestation of sexuality in the subject, in the child, in the constitution of the unconscious. It is in the origin, because sexuality will follow paths, several paths. I think that this is what is important—it begins as masochism, and then one cannot fail to remember it as the *sexual* death drive. These two things are interconnected for Laplanche. I'm going to talk a little about this here, and your questions are mixed. You are asking yourself whether it is possible to get rid of the normative family structures. I think the answer is affirmative. I would also say, I don't know if I would formulate it this way, "to get rid of," because it is what Laplanche is gradually showing. That's to say, it is developing in the theory, which is the place of these structures in the process of the constitution of the sexual unconscious and within the psychic apparatus or the soul.

It is not in the origin. It is not what defines the unconscious, the structure of the unconscious, but instead it's on the side of the mytho-symbolic. The big question for Laplanche is where to topographically locate this, rather than getting rid of the traditional family structures, like Oedipus, for example, as well as others. Laplanche never proposed to abandon these structures. Freud's mistake was to take them as being what is at the origin of the unconscious. What is at the core of the unconscious, that is what Laplanche is going to question. More than masochism, what counts there is the theoretical model that involves the General Theory of Seduction and the translational hypothesis. Masochism seems to be a consequence of all this—almost a point of arrival. It is not enough to exchange one content for another; it is necessary to insert this within a context, which is the General Theory of Seduction and the translational hypothesis. It is a theoretical model that leads him to place masochism as originary, not only as originary but also linked to fantasy. This is the great leap that he will make, in fact so much so that in 1968 he has a text on masochism—a text that he will revisit, revise, and reformulate in 1992.

It's not that he thinks the answers are in philosophy, but he only managed to make a leap, where the ones who helped him make this leap were the philosophers—especially Spinoza. They are going to theorize precisely this question of "the more the knowledge, the more the activity" in the active than in the passive. This, for Laplanche, allows him to introduce the question of fantasy, which is the differential. There is a passage where he says something to the effect of, "For it is the effraction of an excess of message coming from the other that functions as pain. Pain of external origin first and then arising from this internal other that is the repressed fantasy." Then he sees that he is already within the context of the General Theory of Seduction, of the idea that it comes from the other. It is the fantasy of the other that appears as an enigma and that is going to, as we talked about before, disturb all that self-preservative functioning, functioning as equilibrium, as homeostasis.

It is necessary to think about each one of these relations because they go together; to define masochism in the seduction theory, you see that he resorts to fantasy, but not just any fantasy. It is a fantasy constructed from the fantasy of the other, so that the question of the internal and the external is already posed. In other words, that which functions as the basis of sexuality is something that is internal but that came from the outside, and the word "source object" tries to account for this duplicity. Within the General Theory of Seduction, the object that was external is transformed into source—the internal and the external coming together.

I think that this is one of the questions because it refers to the question of autoeroticism that in my understanding Laplanche can't put together; he doesn't manage to integrate this in the body of work. There are, I think, two or three texts in which it is very clear that the emergence of the sexuality that we are talking about, which is masochistic, is also autoeroticism. The first manifestation of sexuality is autoeroticism, and it is masochism at the same time, but he has difficulty in joining these two things, and even less when he goes on to talk about the Third Topographical Model, because I think that is where it was possible to join. In any case, it is also intertwined here; it is all together, as well as the question of on and off. Sexuality has these two sides—it appears as off, it appears as *sexual* death drive, and it is this that will summon something from the child. Something that maybe is genetically or instinctively written. It is the question of the drive to translate, which is José Carlos Calich's work and research interest.

BBT: Without taking us too far astray, you mentioned "the drive to translate." You said it is "the drive." Do you think that perhaps it is an instinct?

LCT: No, he uses the word *pulse* [drive]. Although it is unknown where this *pulse* comes from. He uses the word *pulsion* in French. At the same time, according to Calich, in a personal conversation, Laplanche confessed that he thinks there is something instinctive, and at the same time he agrees that it also depends on the contribution that comes from the adult. But he didn't define how it is constituted. In what Laplanche left published, the drive to translate derives from the message, from the enigmatic. The doubt remains in the air; something is left open. In my understanding, it is necessary to think about both sides, that there is a compromise between an innate tendency and something that comes from outside.

Returning to what we were speaking about previously: The important thing is that from this disconnect, the hermeneutic side of the subject, the ego is activated, and it is the symbolizing side. The side of symbolization, the symbolic path, the translational path is all the mytho-symbolic. The narrative schemes, the complexes: Oedipus, castration complex, etc. Going back to the origin, for him it is not to get rid of the narrative schemes yet. Not even of the traditional ones, because they have a place in the history of the subject. They have a place in the history of culture, and in the topographical level, which is the place of defense, of symbolizing translational movement that serves to deal with and connect the disconnected from the *sexual* death drive. This leads us, in a certain way, to another matter, which is in the question regarding gender.

You include several other matters besides gender: the matters of socioeconomic class, race, etc. But the truth is that Laplanche didn't get very interested in these matters. He restricted himself to dealing with gender, and I believe it was not because he thought those matters were unnecessary or meaningless, but simply because he didn't have time to do it. I think that everything he said about gender could serve as a model for us to think about these other issues. Ideologies have a defensive binding function. All of them in all levels, just as there will be the binary logic, in the question of gender. The binary logic will invade all these other universes, all these other social domains and relationships, not by chance, but because there is a *pulsional* dimension involved.

BBT: Laplanche spoke about gender, and you mentioned that we can use the same structure and thought that he did to think about race, power, class, etc. Can you speak a little more about this?

LCT: Yes, let's get into the discussion of gender; I think it will become clearer later. In "Gender, Sex and the *Sexual*," in *Freud and the* Sexual, there is an attempt to reintroduce the notion of gender in psychoanalysis. In a certain way, he is going to think in this direction from the idea of "identification *by*." He is going to introduce this notion before the child feels identified with the other, he is identified *by* the other. It is something that comes from the social, but it is not from the general social, it is from the small social. He will put gender as coming first; so, there he makes an inversion in the whole sociological discussion, including by Judith Butler and all the feminists and those who discuss gender. He will say, "Well, gender comes first within this idea that it is a designation." He uses this term, gender is "designated"—the child before knowing himself "boy or girl," he is treated, he is named, treated as "boy or girl" by the group of adults. This is what he calls "designation."

He is identified by the other before he identifies himself; but precisely this designation, it is enigmatic, in such a way that this gender comes first. It is plural insofar as it is compromised by the adult's unconscious. Therefore, the adult does not just say, "You are a girl!" The adult is saying more things along with that because the unconscious is passing through in that designation. It is a designation that appears as enigmatic; it is going to require a whole work of symbolization that can be summarized in, "How am I going to identify myself in terms of gender?" But before the "I" of narcissism sees himself this way or that way, he was seen by the other. Now, Laplanche says, "To symbolize, to translate, the child has a binary system ready. A binary narrative scheme that works as a code."

Laplanche will use this social code to translate into masculine and feminine. He uses the word "sex" here. The binary sex, masculine and feminine, serves as a translator, a code that will provide stability, that will give a form to what arrived in an enigmatic way; and the *Sexual* is what is left. It is the residue of this translation. This is the general scheme of that 2003 essay, "Gender, Sex and the *Sexual*." Gender comes first, it is a designation; sex is everything that serves as a code, generally binary, by biological contingency. He says we are divided into male and female by biological contingency. But also, by a social, cultural contingency that was structured around this binary. This is very strong; he says, "Well, this is a code that is present in every culture and that will serve as a translator code." But precisely, he says this binary code is not able to translate the complexity that is the designation of gender because the adult, when he is identifying, he identifies as a boy and a girl, but at the same time as something else. There, it depends on the adult's unconscious. Many times, there is a complex game in the father and mother—a transferential game between them that what is said may not be what one says, as one thing might really be meaning another.

It is not only at the origin but also from the origin—gender is present from the origin as a designation. It is something transversal. It is the same history of the unconscious fantasy of the adult, which is transversal to the plan. Besides being present from the origin, it appears as something that needs to be symbolized. Gender doesn't arrive ready-made; the designation is not finished when we say to the child, "You are a boy!" It's not enough, because what I say and what I do is a little bit scrambled and unclear; it is mixed up with all my unconscious desires, and it demands a symbolization. From this, he says that binarism is one of the forms of connection; there is no doubt, we can say, probably the most efficient. I don't know—or maybe it is also the most defensive in the sense that it has a function of covering up or denying the rest.

It's the whole theory that allows this opening, masochism is one of the points, but there are other points as we are seeing here, like the matter of gender. Gender involves a plurality because of the unconscious, the enigmatic—a plurality that will never be captured. It will be circumvented by a code. The binary code stabilizes, but it stabilizes at the price of repressing the disconnected elements. The binary code serves as an identifying stability, but it's provisional. I think that's how we must think: Something is lost of the enigmatic involving gender that can come back at any moment, and that will force the symbolization process all the time. Going back to this question of normative structures: They have a function. But that is what he will question: "What is important is how well the structure is able to bind." It produces a stability to the extent that it binds, regardless of what structure it is.

But Laplanche also says, "When Freud discusses, for example, the classic text on Leonardo, he is led to speak of a sublimation that is written in the origin before repression." This is what Laplanche will call it; he says, "It needs to be named; this is precisely what we need to think about that is inscribed in the process but is not subjected to repression and will give rise to a movement of symbolization, tied to the enigmatic, to what came from the other." He uses the idea of inspiration because he talks about how inspiration comes from the other, it comes from outside, it's in third person. Laplanche speaks about inspiration as the creative pole of sublimation. Whereas there is a more repetitive pole, which he also calls a symptomatic pole, a repetitive symptom. A more open pole, which is the creative pole. One that is the return of the repressed, and the other that feeds on the enigma before repressing. It is the enigma that inspires. The enigma of the other. But it is the *Sexual* at the same time. It is the *Sexual* producing in this movement.

I don't know if it is possible to retrieve from this the other questions that you had raised, the social questions, the questions about race. It seems that perhaps starting from this discussion about gender, it is possible to think about these other fields in this sense. Perhaps precisely from the idea of sublimation, which connects with the idea of the hermeneut within us, allows in these movements, something of the most symptomatic order or something of the most creative order. When he speaks of the hermeneut, it is this need to symbolize. It is the need to find codes, to seek new translations. It is a process that never ends because of seduction. He always says, "In the same way that in the beginning there was the effraction of the enigma of the other that came from the outside, this effraction will continue coming from the source object"—then always demanding a work of symbolization. Why? Because in the conception of realism that we have seen, this object is never exhausted because it is a signifier of a meaning. It was lost from the hermeneutic universe, it was lost from the semantic universe, the semiotic universe; it went astray. It became a thing. It can never be found again; it is very similar to Lacan's *objet petit a*—it is that which always escapes. It will always repeat an excitation, a suffering that is masochistic in nature.

BBT: Do you think there are holes or incongruencies in Laplanche's work?

LCT: I would identify three major shortcomings or limitations. The first I would say that is most lacking in the work are reflections on the clinical situation. Similarly, the second is that there is also a lack of development on the ego; Laplanche doesn't have a specific text dedicated to the ego. It is dispersed in several texts, although he has a theory on the ego. The third is a certain lack of development, of more depth about the Third Topographical Model and about the theory of *clivage* [splitting].

I think that there are more insufficiencies in the work, but for me these are the central ones, and they are the ones where I was able to make some contributions, like my work on psychosis, for example. I think there is a big gap in Laplanche discussing clinical material. Perhaps we could say that this is the most criticized point in Laplanche's work. But I would say, most of the time, in an unfair way. Unfair due to a misunderstanding of Laplanchean thought itself and starting from a logic that is often inductivist, deductive. Psychoanalysis is founded from the beginning on an inseparable relationship between theory and practice. The analytic method, which is practice, is then inseparable from its object, which is the sexual unconscious.

One of Freud's first confusions was trying to reduce the unconscious to neurosis, hysteria, and even believing at that moment that it was possible for you to be able to overcome this problem. To analyze the unconscious to the end and subvert the whole process. I would say then that in this sense, what is most lacking in Laplanche's work is psychopathology, in the strict sense of psychopathology. Laplanche's great concern was always to reconstruct psychoanalytic theory, metapsychology to explain above all the constitution of the sexual unconscious of the drive [*pulsion*], an unconscious and a sexuality that is universal. As an epistemologist and as a philosopher, he was concerned about: "If psychoanalysis is to sustain itself, it needs awareness that it must have an object that is universal, not one that is specific." Therefore, he is always concerned about whether the sexual unconscious is present in everybody. This is what first needs to be explained. Psychopathology is secondary. It is a consequence of something. It is specific and contingent. The sexual unconscious is not; it is structural, it is universal. If we can explain the constitution of the sexual unconscious, then we can explain how psychopathology is formed. Here is where the big flaw comes in—he didn't commit himself to try to do this.

But the focus is around this more universal clinical practice matter and not around psychopathology. Not that psychopathology is totally absent from his work. It would not be wrong to say that either, but it is true that it is marginal to his work. When he needed to work on psychopathology, he did it through the Freudian cases mainly. He doesn't bring his own clinic, in the broader sense at least, to think about psychopathology. It appears more to discuss some important concepts, for example, angst.

To sum up, it is true, we can say, that there is a certain gap in Laplanche's work regarding the clinic. But contrary to what people think, I would say, I don't believe that this is a problem for the theoretical foundations that he proposes because these foundations aim to explain the universal side—which is the constitution of the unconscious and this clinic.

My personal contribution to filling this gap was my doctoral dissertation on paranoia. The dissertation was published with the title of *Paranoïa et théorie de la séduction généralisée* [Paranoia and the General Theory of Seduction]. I would say that this work came to fill, in part, this gap or part of this gap, one could say here with a double function. On the one hand, launching a look at psychopathology from the General Theory of Seduction, and on the other hand, trying to validate the translational hypothesis to also think about the field of psychoses. It had a double function in this sense, because the matter of psychoses had not entered consideration in a certain way in Laplanche's reflection until the '90s.

BBT: He has that book *Hölderlin and the Question of the Father*, published in 1961, in which he analyzes Hölderlin, who suffered with psychosis.

LCT: Yes, a text that he forgot about because it is still very much bound to Lacanian theory. It was his doctoral dissertation directed by Lacan. Laplanche hardly ever mentioned this text. When he mentioned it, it was to say that it was an initial Lacanian moment. Psychosis remained distant from his reflections. In 1990, he wrote that very short essay called "Implantation, Intromission," in *The Unfinished Copernican Revolution*. This is the first answer he gives to account for the absence of psychosis in his work.

It is as if he had developed the translational model starting from neurosis and had left psychosis aside. We can say Laplanche had already opened the doors to this undertaking with this text, because it was written there to show, or at least to raise the hypothesis, that the translational model serves to think about both neurosis and psychosis: the neurotic psychic life from implantation, and psychosis from intromission. He introduces the notion of intromission to think that messages that come, in a certain way, block the symbolization process, the translation process. Instead of demanding a translation or encouraging the translation, in intromission, what is missing is enigma, and instead of stimulating translation, what we generally have is something that comes to block. The block will give rise to *enclaves,* psychotic *enclaves,* as is the case, for example, with the superego.

I think there are two big questions there that need to be answered, that my work tried to bring a reflection on: First, is the nature of these messages; what kind of messages are these? Second, the status of the *enclaves* that are produced from the blockade; how are these *enclaves* constituted; and what place do they occupy in the topography of the psyche, etc.?

First, I will discuss the nature of these messages and then talk about the status of the *enclaves*. There are paradoxical injunctions that happen in intromission. These injunctions go against enigma, in the sense that Laplanche gives this concept. "Enigma" is based on a signifier of meaning that only communicates an intention to communicate to someone. Going further, most importantly is that enigma is *without* content. The paradoxical injunctions are direct orders with full meanings, but unrelated, and require responses or attitudes that cancel each other out in one's mind. It seems that they are two things exactly that go against each other.

This led me to propose that the paradoxical constitutes the reverse of the enigmatic, in the sense that it is not quite the opposite, or not only the opposite. The reverse is that which is part of, has a continuity. When sexuality is refused, foreclosed by parents, by the adult, it tends to take the form of the paradoxical, that is, it can only be not being. Because that is the essence of the paradoxical—you are not being. And when you are not, you are. If enigma presents itself as not being connected, the paradoxical presents itself with an absolute connection that cannot be undone. But this connection does not cease to be sexual; that is the leap that needs to be made. I would say, the paradoxical intends to exclude the sexual, and it does it in a radical way, and that is by trying to place it on the plane of the self-preservative or reducing it to the self-preservative. The sexual cannot be transformed into self-preservative, so it continues to be sexual, but presented in another way and in an absolute manner. It has no room for questioning, doubt, and ambiguity. This is the greatest mark of psychosis; the delirium is a construction that does not allow for being deconstructed in any way.

This is the greatest obstacle psychosis presents for psychoanalysis, I would say. It is not the transference, contrary to what Freud initially supposed. For Freud, the psychotic individual did not transfer. After Klein, it was discovered that it is just another kind of transference; contrary to the absence, perhaps it is a massive transference in question. It is less the absence of transference that is the obstacle, because in fact there is an obstacle to analysis. But the obstacle is not in the absence of transference; it is more in the fact that the delirium does not allow itself to be deconstructed. This massive transference is also an obstacle because sometimes it completely denies you, it silences, it has this function—as if the other person wasn't there. Transference also constitutes an obstacle, but it's a lesser obstacle than the rigidity of the delirium, and more than that, I would say. Most of the time the condition of transference, the possibility of the existence of transference in psychosis, depends precisely on how much the analyst can respect the delirium. You can never just make your way with a flying kick.

Freud says, "Every delirium has a foundation of truth." It is from this perspective that we need to think about a method, because if you put yourself in this position, different from saying to the psychotic that everything is nothing but a mere fantasy, a mere construction of his head, without any relation to the world. Because if you put yourself in this position, there is no way out, that is, you completely disqualify any possibility of transference. As Laplanche says, it is as if you cut the branch on which you are sitting. You become psychotic; you say, "All this is nothing but a construction in your head. I own the truth and I need to show you that, then you are delirious." If we place ourselves within this perspective that has a real foundation, the persecution translates something of a lived experience, then we open a channel for transference.

The other question is that of the status of the *enclaves* that are produced in the absence of translation, of symbolization. That's my area of study—the paradoxical injunctions are going to give way to *enclaves* in the psyche. My hypothesis there was that these *enclaves* are situated at the level of the superego. As soon as they appear in the delirium, at least in paranoia, the one who attacks is above all the superego, this archaic superego, this more *pulsional* superego.

Even because Laplanche himself already considers the superego as an *enclave*. Sort of following this path, I suggested that the *enclaves* in paranoia tend to situate themselves in the plane of the superego. The question that was left open is a topographical status. With the new theory of *clivage*, in which

Laplanche situates the superego on the side of the *enclaves*. It is necessary to reopen this discussion a little.

It was Christophe Dejours who came up with the idea of the topic of *clivage*. Laplanche also had in his mind the work of Marta Rezende Cardoso, whose doctoral dissertation was about the superego. It followed his indication of the superego as an *enclave*. Cardoso will develop, go far in this direction, and I think Laplanche also had in his mind this work that I did on paranoia, on the psychoses—that is, the idea that it was necessary to consider a psychic space within the psychic structure, a space beyond the superego.

The *enclave* is not loose in the topography. There is a space, a whole enclosing space, which needs to be thought of in a structural way. The other question linked to this is: What is the nature and status of the energy that is linked to *enclave*? As for sexuality, what kind of drive is there? We know that Laplanche didn't develop this because what he wrote on the topic of *clivage* is very programmatic, very reduced, schematic.

Dejours had already proposed, before Laplanche adhered to this model, that this is the realm of the death drive. He doesn't call it an *enclave*; that was Laplanche's choice. Dejours calls it "amential"; and there the death drive is situated, he says, in the Freudian sense and not in the Laplanchean sense, that is, it is not the *sexual* death drive. It is a drive in the sense of instinct. It is the biological drive that became deadly—the biological drive that was not encompassed exactly by the sexual drive and became deadly. This idea for Laplanche doesn't fit, it doesn't make sense, and for me it doesn't make sense either. Everything that happens in this *clivage* space, in this stuck space, is already of the order of the sexual. I would say it like this, much less of the Freudian death drive, and more of the *sexual* death drive; that is, it is the most disconnected sexuality—I would say, connected to the *enclaves* even properly to the superego and to other *enclaves* that form this space.

I am now going to speak about the other two, which are related to the development of the ego and the deepening of the third topography, the topic of *clivage* [splitting]. Let me start by talking about Laplanche's contributions on the ego. From my point of view, I would highlight three major contributions of Laplanche's thought in this respect:

First, Laplanche dwelt on this issue a fair amount in the beginning of his work. His sense of showing that there are not two egos, a metaphorical and a metonymic one, as a certain reading of his work showed. He wrote then a text to respond to that saying that it was a mistake, because, in fact, for him it's about the junction of two derivations. Freud himself had already described those derivations, not with those terms, but according to Laplanche's interpretation, in modern language, it could be called a metonymic derivation, representing the vital, the self-conservative, and together with it, the body. This derivation is soon colonized and dominated by the metaphoric derivation, representing the identifications and then the sexual drive, once the identifications are inscribed in the plane of object relations.

For him, it is not about two egos, but the junction of two derivations that will form an ego, an ego with two tendencies: Where the metonymic tendency is quickly covered, dominated, and colonized by the metaphoric derivation, that is, by the identifications.

BBT: Pardon, in which book or which text does Laplanche say that?

LCT: The first discussion is in *Life and Death in Psychoanalysis*. He returns to make this clarification in a text that was not published. We published it in the book *Entre Sedução e Inspiração: Como Situar o Eu na Obra de Jean Laplanche* [Between Seduction and Inspiration: How to Situate the I in the work of Jean Laplanche], whose title is: "Acerca da minha concepção do Eu" [About my conception of the Self]. It's a manuscript that Laplanche distributed at the university. It's now published in Portuguese. There's no French publication.

This is what Laplanche explored the most and what is most consolidated in his reflection. It culminated in the idea that narcissistic identifications are one and the same thing. This means that the metaphorical derivation is the most important in this process of the constitution of the ego since, according to him, another narcissism than the love for oneself does not exist—a love that is constituted in the wake of the love dispensed by the object. Laplanche said that the idea of Lacan's mirror stage remains, for him, a great inspiration. The "I" is constituted from the identification process that has the other as the center. That is, narcissism for him is inserted in this line of metaphorical derivation, not metonymic.

Another important contribution that Laplanche made, despite all the criticisms that he had about the Freudian idea at the end of his work, was that narcissism would be present from the beginning in a closed, biological state. Laplanche severely criticized the way Freud rethought the concept of narcissism. For Laplanche, the most important text is Freud's "On Narcissism: An Introduction" (1914), where narcissism is the result of a process. It comes with the identifications. It is not present from the beginning. It is a result. Laplanche takes up Freud's phrase in this text, where Freud says, and I paraphrase, "I must admit that there is no such thing as the ego within the psyche. The ego is the result of a process that exists from the beginning." According to Freud, autoeroticism. But narcissism needs a new "psychic action" to exist—this is Freud's term. Therefore, the constitution of narcissism and the ego as an instance are correlative. This is the idea that Laplanche also maintained until the end.

In my opinion, Laplanche's third great contribution to this matter is to have shown that narcissism does not represent only a moment of unification of autoeroticism, that is, of partial drives. This is Freud's central thesis, and Laplanche added that, beyond this unification, narcissism is also inserted in a movement of self-centeredness and closure. This is the other important mark of his reflection on the ego, and it constitutes one of the central theses of the text "The Unfinished Copernican Revolution," in the book of the same title. It is there that he best treated this question. Laplanche said that the function of the initial decentering that he calls Copernican, the child revolving around the adult, is compared to the Ptolemaic, which is an inevitable consequence of narcissistic centering.

I would say that this axis of ego narcissism, this axis of centering, has been little explored so far, and I would say that it is also necessary to think about this self-centering, this movement of self-centering and closing together along with the process of translation, symbolization, which is an eminently active process. It is necessary to think about the whole question of the passage from initial passivity to activity.

In my understanding, this question of self-centering, of closure, and this passage from passivity to activity, needs to be thought of within the topic of *clivage* that constitutes Laplanche's contribution, which was looser in his work, more open, we could say unfinished. It is something that remained more as a project, a model.

A little of my contribution comes in the wake of the discussion, trying to make a dialogue that practically did not exist between Laplanche and Dejours in this respect. My last reflections have been centered around this matter of *clivage* because the introduction of this topic demands the reconsideration, in my understanding, of the whole topography, including the ego topography, which Laplanche didn't do. He adheres to the idea of the third topography, but he doesn't return to the theory and rethink it.

In my understanding, what is at the center of this splitting, functioning there as a kind of structural refusal, is the superego. This thesis I have been defending for some years now. How did I arrive at this hypothesis? What led me to believe that was that the superego is formed through the early interdictions against infantile autoeroticism and thus occupies a frontier position within the topography, separating that which went through the process of translation and repression from that which is refractory to this process.

Laplanche will situate this *pulsional* superego within the topography of *clivage*. That is, in *enclaved* unconscious. Why can we say that it works as a structural refusal? By the way, this is another matter, because Laplanche says that it is necessary to think here about the concept of refusal. He goes back to Freud and says essentially that it is as if there were already indications in Freud that he is not only talking about a specific defense mechanism of perversion, of psychosis, but as something already structural. This is how Laplanche imagines the notion of refusal should be understood.

The splitting for Laplanche is between what has been translated and what has not been translated. That is why I put as the central issue and the issue of otherness the issue of passivity/activity. But why does it function as a structural refusal? I will make an entire discussion saying that maybe we must go beyond the mechanism of refusal.

The definitions that we have of the original repression are always that it is a failure of translation. There is no force in its origin, and here Laplanche is, in my understanding, stuck to Freud. The force is for translation, which comes from enigma. It is enigma that mobilizes the child to translate, and repression is that which could not be translated.

I have to say that this idea bothered some people. I think that the main one was Silvia Bleichmar. She was the one that radically diverged from Laplanche, precisely because she felt the need for an engine for repression and, for her, this engine comes from outside. In this respect, I tend to agree with her. I think that the idea of the failure is still valid. However, it seems to be more the case in the first translations that give origin to autoeroticism. Here is another important point, because although Laplanche theorized about autoeroticism and its relation to repression, this was also left loose in his work.

When he synthesizes, defines the original repression, for example, in the *New Foundations for Psychoanalysis,* he doesn't integrate this question of autoeroticism in repression. However, there are passages, in *Problématiques III: La Sublimation*, where he explicitly describes that repression must have a direct relation with autoeroticism, and that the source-object is already formed there at that moment. It is funny because you read this with a clarity, with a precision, but it gets a little loose, it gets a little lost in the lesson. My hypothesis is that Laplanche couldn't make this bridge because the topic of *clivage* was missing. I think this is as if he didn't know what to do, where to situate the autoeroticism topographically.

BBT: When you say that he didn't know where to place autoeroticism, you are speaking about which decade of his work?

LCT: I think it is missing in all his work. Because he doesn't do this bridge, whenever he is going to define the canonical classic texts about repression, he doesn't deal with autoeroticism. He will relate autoeroticism and repression in a text like sublimation. But this is my hypothesis. This is a reading.

BBT: But it is important.

LCT: Yes. When he incorporates the idea of the third topography, I think that he needed to review many things. One of them is this matter of repression, the relation with autoeroticism. I'm going to propose this departure. I think then, for example, the question of failure seems to me more pertinent to think about in regard to this first translation. There are two passages basically—one is in the text about sublimation, where he considers autoeroticism as a first translation. I am saying, well, I think that this first translation is made in a more spontaneous way. Without the intervention of the adult, without interdiction. Because the interdiction comes later, it comes precisely because this autoerotic translation will put the adult in an uncomfortable position. This autoerotic translation of the child makes the adult disconcerted; it messes with the child's unconscious.

Then the adult will "demand" that the child find another translation. I say that when it is a matter of translating autoeroticism in a new translation, in narcissistic terms, the interdictions of the adult also come into play. In fact, it is these interdictions that drive a new translation and that place a restriction in relation to autoeroticism. But it happens, as it is driven by the censorship of the adult who does not tolerate the autoerotic translation made by the child. This led me to divide the original repression into two times. Laplanche already speaks of two times because it is the theory of *après-coup*. But when he mentions the two times, it is to speak about implantation and the translation. I am saying it is necessary to think one more time, and he himself says this in one or two passages; he adds the expression at least two times.

BBT: In which text?

LCT: This is, for example, in a note in the text "The Drive and Its Source-Object: Its Fate in the Transference," in *The Unfinished Copernican Revolution* (Laplanche & Thurston, 2020, p. 307). He mentions at least twice.[1] I am running with this idea. First, there is the translation into autoeroticism—these are the first translations that the child manages to make that are eminently corporal translations. They happen in a more spontaneous way on the part of the child, but they already involve a failure and a loss. Laplanche himself describes this in that text that I told you about sublimation, and it is the reference to the other, that is, the author of the message. He says, there is already a repressing of the other—that's the expression he uses.

Now, in the second time, we must think then of repression, when the translation of autoeroticism and narcissism takes place. This completes the process of the original repression and then culminates with the beginning of *clivage* and the constitution of the instances. Because in the first time, there was not yet a *clivage*. Autoeroticism doesn't need an "I" in this instance. Autoeroticism happens through the initiative of the body-self, which already translates. Because it doesn't need so many symbolic codes to translate, it is translating more with the body. The second time, a failure is also produced, another loss linked more to the content of the message there, the content that was enriched with the autoerotic fantasy. To constitute autoeroticism, it needs a fantasy still rudimentary, not very symbolic, but it has a fantasy. Then with that which accompanies the interdiction of the adult, because by interdicting autoeroticism, in a certain way the adult is also naming that activity as sexual.

Then I say, the content is enriched, and in this second stage of repression, there will be a loss of the most significant content. While in the first stage, the loss is more related to the object that has become high. The excitement takes place in one's own body, independent of the other. In the new translation, in the second step of the translation, besides this reference to the other being lost, it is also a reference to the content. Because the autoerotic code cannot pass to the other side, the autoerotic code must stay behind. My hypothesis here is that you need the topic of *clivage* because the first translation takes place in the body-self. There is a fixation in the body-self, in this place that will later become the *enclaved* unconscious, in my understanding.

In the second time of that original repression, the fixation happens in the repressed unconscious, because there is already the beginning of the topographical division, and this is very important for the whole process of constitution of the *sexual* life drive. Because the *sexual* life drive needs this fixation. But the source-object has already started in the first time, because that is how Laplanche thinks in this passage. In *New Foundations for Psychoanalysis,* he said that the source-object is constituted from the signifier of meaning, inside the repressed unconscious. In this passage of the text about sublimation, he says that the source-object begins with the constitution of autoeroticism. It implies a duplication of the object. It joins the object of the fantasy related to the other, to milk, etc., and an object that is taken in the body itself, a part of the body. He says this duplication of the object is what gives rise to the source-object. For me, it is the clearest, most important text of the constitution of the drive, and it is the *sexual* death drive. It is constituted as disconnection. It is a disconnection that is not total because it is fixed to the body and is fixed to a fantastical object; but within a logic of partial object, of partial drive, and the logic of the pleasure principle, for him it is the *sexual* death drive—the beginning of the drive.

It is necessary to think that the object is already constituted before the constitution of the repressed unconscious. It is constituted there in the body-self; then in the second moment, this source-object will be fixed in the repressed unconscious. Then this is the point that I say it is necessary to put Laplanche to work and that in my understanding is only possible within the context of the topic of *clivage*.

I was saying earlier that the superego is at the center of the *clivage,* playing the role of separation and functioning with a structural refusal. The big question is to explain how this happens. The refusal always involves two sides: One that affirms and another that denies. The big question here is to know what needs to be denied. In Freud, it is castration, in the real sense; the whole Freudian discussion is centered around the idea of castration—this idea that Lacan will take up again and will reformulate in symbolic terms. Lacan also has a refusal, and it is castration in the symbolic sense.

My hypothesis is that in this development that I propose, starting from Laplanche, what needs to be refused is alterity—is the other in me and all that this represents in the sense of passivity. For me, this is where it is situated, this is where the question of *clivage* is justified. This base of the superego is linked to the first interdictions of autoeroticism. I would say this is at the top of the alterity that needs refusal, this negation. It's at the top because they are the junctions, the interdictions that come from the outside that can't be moved or translated.

I am working with the idea that the refusal happens in two stages as well. The first comes with the constitution of narcissism itself and of the ego, which happens in the second stage of the original repression, when the translation of autoeroticism into narcissism happens. As I said, narcissism represents for Laplanche a closure. We can also add that it is a closure in relation to the external other, but also in relation to the internal other that has in the figure of the superego its main representative. It is necessary to work on Laplanche's text—to say that it is closure, but also a change of position from passivity to activity. Narcissism already represents this—the second stage comes with the constitution of the ideal of the self, which is the double of the superego.

Freud would say that the paradox of the superego exists. It has two sides, a more *pulsional* [drive] side, more archaic; and it has a more evolved side, more symbolic. For me, it is the superego that is inside the *enclaved* unconscious and the ideals that are there in the ego plane. Here, it is necessary, in my understanding, to take up again the idea already present in Freud, that I am talking about the double inscription superego: one more functional and more disengaged, and another more rational and more engaged. It's interesting to remember that Freud affirms this in his text "On Narcissism: An Introduction," where he says that when the narcissistic investment that was deposited in them is taken away from the ideals, the otherness origin of that instance reappears with everything, including persecution.

I really like this passage by Freud because it seems that he anticipates much of what is being discussed here. Because first he will say that narcissism cannot endure. It must stay behind; it must be repressed. But he says nothing disappears in the life of the soul. Narcissism takes refuge in ideals, Freud says. He says it's easy to identify when this narcissistic investment is withdrawn—these internal objects, these ideals, regain the otherness that they possessed in the beginning. For me, he's talking here about two sides of the superego, and I'm proposing that this narcissistic investment of the ideals on the ego plane plays a central role in the constitution of the structural refusal that sustains the vertical *clivage*. And, for me, it's the *clivage* between what came from the outside and what remains of the other in the form of otherness, including the superego.

Note

1 "This, then, is where we need to discuss originary repression. For it is in a single process that such repression both splits off a primordial unconscious from the psyche (which thereby *becomes* an id) and constitutes the first source-objects, the sources of the drive. In accordance with the Freudian theory of *après-coup*, I conceive of originary repression as having at least two stages."

Bibliography

Freud, S. (1914). On narcissism: An introduction. In J. Strachey (Ed. & Trans.), *The standard edition of the complete psychological works of Sigmund Freud* (Vol. 14, pp. 67–102). Hogarth Press and the Institute of Psycho-Analysis.

Laplanche, J. (1980). *Problématiques III: La sublimation*. PUF.
Laplanche, J. (2011). *Freud and the sexual*. The Unconscious in Translation.
Laplanche, J., & Carson, L. (2007). *Hölderlin and the question of the father*. ELS Editions.
Laplanche, J., & House, J. (2016). *New foundations for psychoanalysis*. The Unconscious in Translation.
Laplanche, J., & Mehlman, J. (1976). *Life and death in psychoanalysis*. Johns Hopkins University Press.
Laplanche, J., & Mehlman, J. (2015). *Between seduction and inspiration: Man*. The Unconscious in Translation.
Laplanche, J., Nicholson-Smith, D., & Marcello, B. (2015). *The temptation of biology: Freud's theories of sexuality*. The Unconscious in Translation.
Laplanche, J., & Thurston, L. (2020). *The unfinished Copernican revolution: Selected works, 1967–1992*. The Unconscious in Translation.
Tarelho, L. C. (1999). *Paranoïa et théorie de la séduction généralisée*. PUF.
Tarelho, L. C., Laplanche, J., Carvalho, M. T., Andrade, F., Belo, F., Balvé Behr, K., Lattanzio, F., Carvalho, I. S., Ribeiro, M., De Carvalho Ribeiro, P., De Ulhôa Cintra, E. M., & Calich, J. C. (2022). *Entre sedução e inspiração: Como situar o eu na obra de Jean Laplanche*. Zagodoni Editora.

6 José Carlos Calich

Sociedade Psicanalítica de Porto Alegre, Porto Alegre, Brazil

Bryan Batista-Thomas: In a previous conversation, you expressed an interest in epistemology. If I may ask, could you say more?

José Carlos Calich: I think epistemology is fundamental to understanding human thinking. It is the discipline that studies the origin of knowledge, the justification for its fundaments, the discussion about the assumptions or assumption systems that underpin it, its limits, and paradoxes, as well as the notion of truth that each system of thought originates. I've been studying epistemology for years in different places and contexts, and I have been participating in conferences on mainly psychoanalytic epistemology. Because I have been an associate editor of the *International Journal of Psychoanalysis*, I had to take this seriously because if you cannot have a reading that is based on epistemology, probably most of the time, you're going to be captured by culture and its trends. You can find in Laplanche's papers that it was at the center of his method.

BBT: What you mentioned previously regarding "thinking in the right path" as it relates to psychoanalytic epistemology sort of makes me think of Laplanche's conception of "going astray"—where Freud went astray. I'm curious how you see that, theoretically and clinically, as it relates to Laplanche's work.

The other thing that I thought was very interesting was that you used your understanding of the mytho-symbolic to understand culture. In some ways, it sounds like there's an expansion that's happening in your thinking as it relates to the mytho-symbolic, or thinking

DOI: 10.4324/9781032670287-7

that you're doing in terms of the mytho-symbolic. Perhaps a separation in terms of epistemology and the mytho-symbolic, if I'm understanding correctly. Could you draw that out and separate it a little bit more?

JCC: The isolated expression "thinking in the right path" is a source of misunderstanding. It could mean there is only one way of thinking. What I was referring to was precisely about epistemology and the necessity of understanding the origins of concepts and their articulation on a new theory or the modification or expansion of an old one. It is related to the coherence with the foundations of a theory. In general, a good new theory, or even an expansion of a current one, is an "epistemological leap," not moving astray, as Laplanche mentions.

On this subject, Laplanche said repeatedly that he didn't want to develop anything clinically before the theory was solid enough to be considered a clinical development of the theory and not a practical engagement of the clinical space with the theory. Because, he said, doing it like that, as many theories have done, makes the theory weak—it does not sustain over time. His idea was that the theory must be intensely solid to then develop something clinical. Laplanche has very few papers that mention anything clinical. Everything we can say about clinical Laplanche are thoughts derived from his theory of technique that he mentioned in his papers or discussions, the personal discussions we had with him. What can help us is trying to follow his epistemological thinking and trying to apply that to the methodology he uses in the fragments of clinical thinking. Otherwise, it would be something that, as Laplanche forcefully expresses with the term "going astray," he firmly rejected the idea that psychoanalysis involves hermeneutics. According to Laplanche, psychoanalysis is not a form of hermeneutics and cannot be grounded solely in metaphysics.

That is where some of the so-to-say Laplanchean developments are going at this moment. They do not follow Laplanchean methodology. They do not follow the importance of the *Sexual*, the message, and mainly, its translation in the center. They do not follow the theory he created about how sexuality is the center of the human psyche. I think this is important and singular in Laplanche's thinking that, if you understand that, hermeneutics becomes something that is completely astray. Otherwise, I think it is very complicated to give a "Laplanche view about clinical work" because he has not published anything systematic about it. But he has given some hints, consistent ideas about the process, some ideas about transference, the idea about *refusement*,[1] and this is published.

BBT: What constitutes a Laplanchean *style* of psychoanalysis?

JCC: It's quite challenging to use certain adjectives because when we try to describe a style, adjectives are essential. I find it particularly difficult to use adjectives to encapsulate what Laplanche thinks about psychoanalysis. It's important to grasp the nuances rather than rely on an adjective that oversimplifies everything. In our use of adjectives, we must avoid what today might be considered biased or prejudicial thinking.

When you use adjectives, you're already imposing a category that must either be accepted or rejected, which is different from understanding the process, the method, or the journey. It's an entirely different approach to exploring how sexuality contributes to the development of the psyche of a person. This is not the same as applying an adjective that, in some way, labels something as good or bad, acceptable or unacceptable.

If I had to describe Laplanche's style, I would likely begin by calling it an intensely rigorous methodology. That would be my first choice of adjectives. I believe his style is rooted in epistemological thinking and rigorous methodology, as well as his understanding of sexuality from its inception—the primal force that shapes the human being from within, the human being in the human.

BBT: The "human being in the human"?

JCC: Although it is not written in detail, Laplanche, in *New Foundations for Psychoanalysis*, considers the psyche as an emergent property. To my understanding, seeing the psyche as an emergent property suggests that it somehow separates from natural biological evolution. This emergence creates a new realm, a new way of relating. However, I believe it must be understood as something that arises from biology, from the body, and forms a new space with its own unique properties.

This, I think, is central to Laplanche's style. He consistently connects the body and mind, but in a distinct way. He precisely defines the realms of the body and the psyche and explains how they relate. This is ultimately an epistemological issue. When we speak of a complex structure like the psyche—an extraordinarily intricate system—we are referring to different realms with distinct properties that interact. This doesn't mean there are no differences; rather, it means there are various interrelated dimensions. The variables and elements are all present.

Here's an example that might clarify the idea: When discussing the analyst and the analysand, the analyst is a system and an individual. That individuality is not self-contained; it interacts. The analyst has his own history, personality, thoughts, experiences of repression, foreclosures, and sexuality. This individuality shapes and produces their own psyche.

The patient follows a similar path. Here, we have two individualities that interact, and through this interaction, they create a new relational space. However, this doesn't mean the distinct individualities simply vanish. It's not that we were once one, then two, and now through our relationship, we become three, four, or five. Rather, the relationship creates multiple spaces, not just one.

BBT: Is this psychic reality the reality of the message and dimensions of that?

JCC: The message, particularly sexual messages, stimulates a need for translation. This is at the heart of Laplanche's idea and the process of metabolization—a transformation (metabole) that occurs with the message, turning something unfamiliar into something that can be integrated within the self. This concept of *metabole* involves a change that produces something recognizable, something that becomes a part of you. It can be compared to digestive metabolism, where a substance is transformed to be recognized and absorbed (integrated) by the organism. I believe this idea is central to Laplanche's thinking, as, to my reading, he consistently emphasizes an intense economic dimension throughout many of his works. The foreign element creates an economic imbalance because, being sexual, it excites the body. This excitement disturbs the system, and the body must find a way to restore equilibrium (homeostasis).

In my view, this is the central idea, the core. However, understanding the nature of translation introduces another major issue. I believe, and Dominique Scarfone agreed more than once with it, in an idea that I once presented to Laplanche: The translational function is a biological one. It is natural, producing this "neo-code" is part of human evolution. I often disagree with Laplancheans who don't share this understanding, but without it, how can we explain the origin of translational activity? If, as Laplanche suggests, this function gives rise to humanity, it must be universal. It doesn't occur only in specific groups or at varying levels—it is a universal phenomenon, part of the Fundamental Anthropological Situation. If it's an invariant—something that always happens in the relationship between infants and adults—then it must have a biological basis. I can't see any other option but to consider this "Fundamental Anthropological Situation" as an aspect of human evolution and evolutionary anthropology. I believe Laplanche alludes to this in *Après-coup: Problématiques VI*. While he doesn't state it explicitly, perhaps because he couldn't fully affirm it, I asked him if he agreed with me. Laplanche replied, "Yes, but you must write about that." He said, "I don't have time to write, and it's very complicated. You should write about that. But I agree with you."

BBT: What section of *Après-coup: Problématiques VI* are you referencing?

JCC: It's not exactly a section, but it forms part of the conceptual framework. *Après-coup: Problématiques VI* is a book that stands apart from the others. All the *Problématiques* were originally seminars at the University of Paris—Sorbonne Université. Laplanche published each *Problématique* one year after the seminar was held. However, with *Après-coup: Problématiques VI*, it took him seventeen years to publish. In my view, this is not a coincidence. There was something there that he was unsure about, something he had to revisit and refine multiple times before publishing. Otherwise, he would have released it after a year, as with the others. It's unusual for his methodology to involve such an extended period of reflection.

I believe the issue was that he sought to define a clear purpose for the translational activity. He was searching for something concrete to articulate. I think he dropped many hints suggesting that this was the direction he was headed, but he never reached a definitive conclusion. He published *Problématiques VI* because he knew his life was nearing its end.

In "La révolution copernicienne inachevée," Laplanche (2008, p. 330) unequivocally mentions its origin: *"It is equally valid that if analysis aims to undo these imperfect translations presented by the patient—their current life, dreams, symptoms—there must already exist, within human existence in general, an inherent movement of translation, de-translation, and re-translation."* (Free translation from the French by this author. Emphasis added.)[2]

BBT: How do you situate the translational process as being something biological and still stay in fidelity with his theory? Because Laplanche said that Freud went astray with the body, biologizing things.

JCC: What Laplanche argued is that Freud was mistaken in claiming that infantile sexuality is biological. According to Laplanche, it is not—and I agree. Infantile sexuality is a byproduct of a translational activity, a binding function that blends the sexual messages of adults, basic human emotions, and attachment dynamics, with the auxiliary influence (whether supportive or not) of the pseudo-unconscious of the mytho-symbolic, which provides the structure for shaping the creation of meaning. It is not biological. However, in my understanding, the starting point, the origin, the "blender," is a biological activity—a translation function—that every human possesses, which leads to the emergence of a new property: the psyche. This likely explains why, with few exceptions, we all have a psyche that shares common structures and properties (invariants), yet is intrinsically different as we create individual meanings. It's important to note that this emergent property is distinct from cognition, which, in this model, will be affected afterward by the "auto-translational" activity.

BBT: It's sort of like the hardware in some ways.

JCC: Yes, exactly. Once the process of translation begins, meaning starts to emerge. According to my reading of Laplanche, meaning is a byproduct of this activity or function; it is not teleological. As I mentioned, Laplanche agreed with this. What occurred is that the biological need to resolve the imbalance caused by the sexuality of the other required a solution. The solution was the activation of this function, probably

> part of our evolutionary genetics, which generates meaning. Producing meaning signifies that it no longer belongs solely to the other; it becomes *my* meaning. Even when an adult conveys a message to me, I now have my own interpretation of it, one that I've created. Now that it is mine, it plants a root of belonging, of continuity, a perspective of the future, a self that I can call my own, just as Laplanche so often reminds us.

Some might propose different solutions. However, if there are invariants, I can only think that it stems from a biological source rooted in evolutionary theory. We have selected it in Darwinian terms because it represents the survival solution: the activation of a function that incidentally generates meaning. As a result, we became beings capable of producing meaning to our emotional experiences, of the emotional communication of the others. This, as Laplanche put it, is the essence of humanity.

BBT: You just solved a problem that I had with Laplanche's work, which is one that ends up being a sort of the chicken or the egg. How is it that there's implantation and/or intromission of sexuality through the compromised message from the adult and then from that adult's generation above? At a certain point, where does it come from? It is sort of a Darwinian problem too, which is for Darwin, what is the originary species? But the title of his book was *On the Origin of Species*, not the originary species. It is a book about natural selection.

Darwin doesn't necessarily give the initial point. He just gives the evolution of it. But what's interesting about what you're saying is that by biologizing it, you offer a solution to where that initial sexuality comes from. In the Laplanchean sense, it comes through a biological process of the translational process in a human, so thereby, it just arises from that. You sort of give, in a Freudian sense, a bedrock. You solve a dilemma, an inconsistency in Laplanche's work.

JCC: That's exactly what I think. I think you understood me. I'm very glad because people will usually just refuse the idea before understanding that this is solving a dilemma. Then, not only a dilemma but integrating what happened to animal evolution, and the hypothesis is we became humans because we have a mutation, or more than one, in the Darwinian sense. A mutation that is good enough to produce translation, permitting us to survive the disequilibrium with this translational function and inserting us into the human realm. In this complexity, this function produces so many different psychic spaces and spaces to relationships that are not primarily related to biology. Because we produce something new, an emergent property that is outside biology. It came from biology, but now it's a new property. That's why I stressed Laplanche's idea of the emergent property, emergence, which is there in the *New Foundation for Psychoanalysis*.

BBT: I don't know if I would agree. But for now, I do. It's a compelling argument that solves a dilemma in his work.

JCC: I think this is a dilemma that must be resolved. Fantasy is a creation of the translation. The possibility of having meaning creates a new space where, based on the translation of the set of sexual messages, you can create desires, imagine, and fantasize about how to fulfill them. That's where we flow. This is infantile sexuality. That's the reason why Laplanche said this is not biological. This is not related to hormones or the developmental phases that Freud mentions in *Three Essays on the Theory of Sexuality*. This is not related to anything directly connected to biology. It is produced by the creation of meaning by translation. But translating has an origin. This is a new property. The new property is being a human that fantasizes and has the capacity of creating a meaning to what you feel. In my view, Laplanche's model offers a way to create an internal emotional reality and to imagine an external emotional reality, based on an "as if" dynamic (as in an imaginary model).

BBT: The *as if* quality of what? Psychic reality, the understanding of the message?

JCC: Let's begin with perception. Freud believed that the psyche originates with perception, but Laplanche countered, saying, "It's not perception, it's the reality of the message." Perception alone doesn't lead to meaning; it merely creates indexes in the process of semantic development. These indexes are not, and never will be, symbols. There must be something more.

I believe this "something more" refers to a translational ability that allows us to produce meaning *as if*. We don't perceive emotions directly; rather, we come into contact with them. We imagine something coherent with our translations. In imagining something that aligns with our emotional experiences and is consistent with our narrative history, we create a new psychic reality. This is fundamentally different from sensory perception.

BBT: This leads me to how you conceptualize the Fundamental Anthropological Situation and the analytic situation in relation to your understanding of the complexity of the situation, the complexity of the psyche?

JCC: The Fundamental Anthropological Situation is precisely the universal context in which this activity is triggered. Laplanche outlines the key elements in this scenario: the child, the adults, the culture, and the process of translation. My understanding of Laplanche's concept of the Fundamental Anthropological Situation is truly anthropological in the strictest sense of the term. It encompasses society, culture, the individual, and their origins. This situation is essential—without adults, a child cannot become human. In the analytic setting, it is necessary to recreate this Fundamental Anthropological Situation to stimulate the activity of translation.

BBT: I'm curious to know how you conceptualize this.

JCC: There are indeed a few points worth discussing here. Laplanche highlights the importance of dissymmetry, which is crucial because it is dissymmetry that establishes the Fundamental Anthropological Situation in the session. Dissymmetry doesn't imply superiority; it simply means difference. Red will never be blue—it's not about one being superior or the other inferior, but rather that they are distinct. We are not the same, and we cannot be.

The analyst must maintain an analytical stance and a mindset that creates the conditions to reestablish what we call the Fundamental Anthropological Situation. This stimulates the process of translation. It's not a social conversation, nor something natural—this is often difficult because people expect analytic dialogue to feel natural, but it cannot be. It must always be dissymmetrical. This isn't about dominance; it's about difference.

I am always the other. Being the other, I stimulate the one. The other is always an enigma. This enigma stimulates the subject. That's the reason why Laplanche called one of his books *Essays on Otherness*. Because the other always stimulates. What is in the core is the sexual other. The *Sexual other* doesn't mean gender and sexuality; it means the whole complexity of the sexual desires and other paths for the child. The child must translate what's happening to give a meaning to something that just produces excitement. When we are in a relationship with another person, and the person has a series of indefinite sexual excitements, we perceive it in our body. It's not in our mind. We receive it. It doesn't mean sexual, genital sexuality. It means that there is something, there's a force, there is an energy that we receive. We perceive that in our body. We feel it in our skin. It's a skin relationship, because I get closer to that person. It simulates something in my body long before thinking occurs.

I am always the other. By being the other, I can stimulate the person who is in contact with me. The other is always an enigma, and this enigma activates the emergence of a subject. At the core of this concept is the sexual other, though "sexual" here does not refer to gender or genital sexuality alone. It encompasses the entire complexity of sexual desires and other pathways for the child. The child must translate what's happening, assigning meaning to something that initially only generates turbulence and/or excitement.

When we engage with another person, and he experiences a range of indefinite sexual excitations, we sense it in our bodies, not in our minds. We receive this kind of "bodily charge" —it doesn't necessarily refer to genital sexuality. Instead, it is a force, a drive that we absorb, something we feel in our bodies. It's a bodily attunement as we come closer to the other person. This drive stirs something within us long before any conscious thought arises.

This movement is what establishes the Fundamental Anthropological Situation. It's also what must be allowed to happen in an analytic setting. The analysand must experience the analyst as an enigma, which stimulates their own translational activity, helping them produce symbols, meaning, and their expansions. The analyst's role is not to provide meanings, but to stimulate translation so that the analysand can generate their own. This is how a new individuality is created, one that is entirely distinct.

BBT: Pivoting quite a bit: can we speak a little bit about dreams and the General Theory of Seduction?

JCC: I believe that when Laplanche redefined the topographical distribution of the psyche, or soul, he also transformed our understanding of dreams. In dreams, some images are likely shaped by our oneiric activity, which is essentially a process of translation. Meanwhile, other images may emerge directly from the enclaved unconscious.[3] Freud referred to this as the "navel of the dream."

For Freud, this was an exception: those parts of the dream that remain inaccessible to interpretation, originating perhaps from the body or elsewhere. Similarly, in Laplanche's theory, the "*enclaved* unconscious" constitutes a significant part of the unconscious. I believe there are more elements in dreams that function merely as discharge rather than as part of the dream work following translational activity.

BBT: Does this revision capture your intended meaning more clearly? But there are probably differences, meaning that we have some parts of the dream that are without meaning. But in a neurotic person, most of the dreams will have meaning. That is understandable that some parts are without meaning; they're just expressions of the body or the dynamics or pressures. This changes Freud's theory a little.

JCC: It expands the concept of the "navel of the dream" and links it to the *enclaved* unconscious. I believe it's important to distinguish between what occurs when we are awake and when we are asleep. Dreaming can be compared to an act of translation, but I don't think we are always engaged in meaningful thoughts while awake. Instead, I believe there is a fluctuation, an oscillation, between moments of meaning and moments without meaning.

BBT: Could you say a little more about how dreaming activity is connected to translation, and specifically this notion of oscillation?

JCC: Oscillation is an inherent aspect of complexity. It is likely that all psychic processes exhibit an oscillatory dynamic. We can understand narcissism and our relationships with others as a continuous oscillation—constantly shifting between self-focus and attunement with others. We are never exclusively oriented towards ourselves or entirely towards others. As long as we do not fall into a pathological narcissistic structure, we remain capable of moving fluidly between these two states. Although I do not recall Laplanche explicitly using the term "oscillation," the concept is applicable in many contexts when describing his ideas. Even his notion of translation involves translating, de-translating, and re-translating.

Although I don't think Laplanche describes it precisely this way, it is crucial to distinguish cognitive thinking from the kind of thinking that follows translational activity. Cognitive thinking is likely an inherent part of being human, possibly resulting from various mutations in our species' developing brain over millions of years. It is independent of the Fundamental Anthropological Situation and not inherently tied to translational activity. The primary function of psychic space is to generate meaning, which is particularly significant in dreams. Dreams convey meaning when they involve translational processes; however, if they originate from the *enclaved* unconscious, they lack inherent meaning. Likewise, purely bodily functions are devoid of meaning. By paying close attention, it is sometimes possible to recognize certain organic illnesses in dreams—not through their symbolic meaning but through expressions of bodily functions that reflect underlying pathological conditions.

BBT: I'm curious about your thoughts on the clinical vignettes that I sent you, specifically the one where the person has a nosebleed in my office, given that we're talking about the *enclaved* unconscious.

JCC: Some preliminary remarks. I think your vignettes are too brief, which prevents us from getting closer to understanding the patient. Instead, we only get a sense of the specific situation you are describing. It is more of a phenomenon than a means of genuinely connecting with the person. Another issue is the absence of any mention of the history of transference, which I believe is fundamental to psychoanalytic thinking, including Laplanche's approach. For example, in *A Short Treatise on the Unconscious*, included in *Between Seduction and Inspiration: Man*, Laplanche states that Freud's analysis of Leonardo da Vinci could never be considered a genuine analysis or analytic thought because there was no transference involved. Without a history of transference, it is impossible to fully engage with the Fundamental Anthropological Situation, the act, or the enigmatic messages at play.

In one of your vignettes, for example, you mentioned a patient who had accumulated significant credit card debt and was unable to pay for sessions. You explained that the fee was mutually renegotiated but you do not mention that it was analyzed. The unconscious dynamics at play were not explored, even though it was evident that something significant was happening. The patient told you he couldn't afford to pay for the sessions, yet he was able to buy a ring and go on vacations.

I think it's important to recognize that this was a negotiated arrangement, which is a conscious process. You consciously negotiated with the patient, but did not engage with the unconscious meaning behind his communication, particularly his desire to pay less, for whatever reasons. In a Laplanchean context, this is a form of communication tied to a segment of the unconscious. It could indicate that he does not want intimacy or contact with his conflicts or that he has other priorities for his pleasures, limits, and so, money—there are several possibilities. However, his unwillingness to pay is connected to his desire rather than the objective reasons he provided. You mentioned that one day the analysand came into a session stating he was going on a three-week vacation and had bought an engagement ring, despite having said just a few months earlier that he was in considerable credit card debt and needed to reduce the frequency of his sessions.

The focus here is on what was happening between you and the patient. Why did he decide to change the frequency of sessions? Why did he want less contact with you? Transference is essential to understanding his motivations, and if we consider Laplanche, we must center our understanding on the transference. You don't have to agree, but do you understand my point?

BBT: I both agree and understand, and I'll make a comment after regarding that.

JCC: At that moment, the analysand spontaneously experienced a nosebleed. This bleeding also serves as a form of communication—he was likely tense about something repressed, and you had opened the doors of repression. He could have exhibited another symptom, but instead, he had this one, indicating something was wrong with his nose; he bled in front of you. I believe Laplanche would emphasize the significance of frequency—frequency of contact with you, with his unconscious, and with the message—as the central element of this vignette.

BBT: Could you say why?

JCC: My impression from this very brief vignette is that there was something within the transference that made him want to see you less frequently.

BBT: If we think about the Laplanchean conception of transference, would this be more on the level of the hollowed-out transference or of the filled-in transference?

JCC: I believe this represents a "filled-in" transference rather than a "hollowed-out" one. His decision to reduce the frequency of sessions was not a mere discharge or something devoid of meaning; I think it carried significant meaning. Although Laplanche never explicitly wrote about this, other authors have—this is a case of acting-in. It is not acting-out because it takes place within the transference rather than outside of it. There was an underlying desire to avoid seeing you, though I am unsure how many times a week he was attending.

He could not continue coming those times a week, but we lack sufficient material to understand the reason behind this. I find the vignettes to be too phenomenological. We are presented with situations, but without enough focus on transference, I cannot provide insight into the person themselves.

BBT: What I wanted to mention about the transference is when I spoke privately with Hélène Tessier about this case, she mentioned that I was speaking outside the *baquet* [the tub]. I was making an inquiry (my comment on how the analysand was able to pay for the ring and a vacation even though he was in debt and wanting to cut back on sessions) that was on the level of the self-preservative as compared to inquiring more on the level of fantasy.

Udo Hock pointed to something like you did, in terms of the acting-in of the communication. What you said about opening the doors of repression. Udo mentioned someone asking Laplanche, "What is the unconscious?" and his response was, "When you fall and break your leg." In this case, to spontaneously bleed is an example of the unconscious simply coming out, without meaning—it just appears, and there's nothing there.

JCC: However, this lack of meaning does not necessarily indicate that it originates from the *enclaved* unconscious. It simply means that, within this material, we are unable to discern the meaning. This is not a psychosomatic disease; it is a psychosomatic reaction, which is quite different. A psychosomatic disease likely has no inherent meaning from the outset. In contrast, a psychosomatic reaction is like experiencing abdominal pain before an exam or before meeting a boyfriend or girlfriend—this abdominal pain is not a psychosomatic disease; it is a psychosomatic reaction that carries meaning. The bleeding itself is just bleeding, but it holds significance; in a certain way, he was burying something.

BBT: Thinking about failure of translation and intromission, would you conceptualize this as maybe something that was intromitted at some point, which is why he bled?

JCC: No, I think when we talk about intromission, we are referring to a pathology of dissymmetry, where the adult communicates their narcissism in an invasive manner, overwhelming the baby with sexual content. If you were so narcissistic that your sexual content was invading this patient, it could be considered intromission—but I don't think that applies here. In this material, you merely lifted the veil, and he bled. He bled because he was predisposed to bleeding, not because you caused it. To elaborate further, imagine he has a family history of hypertension that has yet to be diagnosed. In this scenario, when you lifted the veil, he experienced a spike in blood pressure due to the exposure, which caused the bleeding. It's usual for individuals with uncontrolled or undiagnosed hypertension to have nosebleeds as a result.

BBT: I'm curious if you felt that any of these vignettes were hollowed-out transference from the information that you have.

JCC: No, not at all. The instance closer to a hollowed-out transference is the one where the analysand reacts with intense rage. With this level of intensity, I believe it already reflects a hollowed-out transference, as it is disproportionate to the situation. What you said should not have triggered such rage—it wasn't about the content of your words. I think they latched onto the phrasing of "you are," interpreting it as creating a separation between themselves and the analyst. They are likely someone struggling to be recognized and deeply afraid of exclusion, with fusion as their solution. They cannot accept that you are different—that you are not the same person—and feel this so strongly that they won't even consider you as a separate individual. After all, what you said wasn't an accusation; it was simply a sentence using "you are," a structure anyone would use. What was the exact quote?

BBT: "Sounds like you're going to have a difficult time when distribution happens."

JCC: Yes, sounds like *you're* going to have a difficult time. They wanted you to say, "We have a problem, and I will be fused with you forever." This reflects the primitive wish of an infant to remain fused, without acknowledging any difference or separation. To me, this appears to come closest to emerging from the *enclaved* unconscious and from a hollowed-out transference.

BBT: The differentiation between when one would recognize the hollowed-out as compared to the filled-in transference is in the intensity of the response not matching the situation itself.

JCC: This is one of the characteristics, but not the main difference.

BBT: Do you mind going over it a little because I haven't read *Problématiques V: Le Baquet. Transcendance du transfert*, as it hasn't been translated into English yet. I will start reading it in Portuguese soon.

JCC: In hollowed-out transference, the associations are not linear; something goes astray. This does not mean there cannot be non-linear leaps, in filled-in transference, but these are typically part of the process. With hollowed-out transference, however, something deviates from the expected path—the patient says something that is outside of linear thinking, even when accounting for leaps, complexity, and expansion. Most importantly, it evokes a deeply unpleasant response in you.

BBT: In me?

JCC: Yes, it evokes something in the analyst that creates an unusual state of mind. Many authors have described this phenomenon. Are you familiar with Michel de M'Uzan?

BBT: Yes.

JCC: De M'Uzan uses the Greek mythological figure Chimera—a creature composed of parts from different animals—to illustrate how the analyst feels in such situations. You find yourself facing something that evokes a sense of discomfort or vertigo, possibly even symptoms in the analyst, such as an interruption of thought, because it is so fragmented that it induces a similar disconnection in you. You listen to the patient and his associations, the free associations that are part of our work, our explorations. Yet there is something that falls outside the map, triggering a reaction in you that feels almost psychotic, evoking a sense of being lost, and primitive anxiety. It is disconnected, unlinked, and induces a disconnection within you—an experience that relates to the *sexual* death drive.

BBT: It makes me wonder if that's Laplanche's understanding of countertransference because he doesn't really have one; he's against the concept. But in that way, within the transference, there's a very specific, almost intersubjective situation.

JCC: The issue here is conceptual, as it involves intersubjectivity and countertransference. Laplanche avoids using the term "countertransference" because he does not consider it to be a form of unconscious communication, a projective identification, and therefore cannot conceptualize it as such. However, he does address the role of the analyst in the session. The analyst's presence and his desires are so significant that Laplanche believes the transference is actively produced by the analyst's presence.

BBT: Are you referencing "Transference: Its Provocation by the Analyst," from *The Unfinished Copernican Revolution*?

JCC: Yes, it's a pity Laplanche did not develop this further, but I am convinced that he deliberately avoided mixing it with concepts like projective identification, unconscious communication, or the intersubjectivity between parent and child. He argued that these ideas were incorrect, yet he did not propose an alternative concept. I don't believe this means he thought these dynamics didn't exist; instead, he simply chose not to conceptualize them in that way within his theory.

BBT: How does one work in the hollowed-out transference, as compared to something that's more filled-in?

JCC: "With filled-in transference, the work involves de-translation and, afterward, re-translation. In hollowed-out transference, the focus is on stimulating the Fundamental Anthropological Situation, shaping the analyst's attitude, and refraining from imposing any meaning (*refusement*), operating not as encouragement but as an impetus that sets psychic work in motion, thereby allowing the patient to produce meaning themselves." The difference between Laplanche and most other psychoanalytic authors (except mainly Lacan, who I believe shares a similar perspective here) is that you do not attempt to interpret meaning where none exists. Lacan would argue that it is pointless to interpret anything symbolically for a person who is not operating within a symbolic register. If the individual is in an imaginary register, interpretation is of no help—it would simply place the interpreter in the role of the "subject supposed to know."

When you interpret something that the patient can only either obey or disobey, there is no opportunity for them to create meaning. Therefore, it becomes essential to foster the production of meaning. One solution, according to Lacan, was to interrupt the session. Laplanche, however, emphasized a different approach centered on the analyst's attitude—by re-establishing the Fundamental Anthropological Situation through a state of *refusement*, which in turn stimulates meaning by activating the translational process.

I asked Laplanche on more than one occasion about Piera Aulagnier, as he mentioned her a couple of times in his work. He said that Aulagnier is someone who must be studied carefully, and so he did. I believe this is because there are structural similarities between their theories.

BBT: Which ones are you thinking of?

JCC: Primarily, metabolization. Before using the term "translation," Laplanche initially used "metabolization" or "metabole." He referred to "metabole" and the "enigmatic signifier." In *New Foundations for Psychoanalysis* and *A Short Treatise on the Unconscious,* included in *Between Seduction and Inspiration: Man,* he discusses his shift to the terms "translation" and "message" and explains his reasons for the change. I believe Laplanche developed an original theory that drew upon the work of those who inspired him—by building on their ideas, starting with Freud, Lacan, Melanie Klein, and, I think, Piera Aulagnier.

BBT: When situating the bedrock of the translational process in biology, do we run the risk of leaving the boundaries of psychoanalysis, given that its object of study is the unconscious? How do you feel that this development in research and thinking remains at fidelity with Laplanche's thinking?

JCC: I believe this is the primary reason why psychoanalysis is sometimes dismissed by other disciplines. It's not only due to prejudice against the ideas but rather a lack of integration—psychoanalysis often struggles to engage in dialogue with other fields, mainly evolutionary genetics. Laplanche often emphasized that a fundamental mistake was to think of infantile sexuality as being solely a product of biology. From the beginning, he argued that this was a misstep in Freud's thinking. In *Three Essays on the Theory of Sexuality*, Freud initially introduced the concept as psychosexual, but as he developed the work, he leaned heavily towards a biological explanation, framing development through distinct stages. Laplanche, on the other hand, proposed that biology needs to be resituated—not eliminated, but placed where it belongs. He emphasizes this strongly yet never denies our connection to biology.

There is a common oversimplification that Laplanche believes all processes originate solely in the body. What he actually means is that the body serves as the original source. Laplanche refers to this in the *New Foundations for Psychoanalysis*, and when, for example, discussing the ego, mentioning that there are various instinctual structures that activate the originary ego (Laplanche, 2021; Tarelho, 2021; Calich, 2021). Although he doesn't fully develop this idea, he explicitly acknowledges it. It is a mistake to think that Laplanche disregards biology at the outset. In the origin, in the Fundamental Anthropological Situation, translation is already present. This is a universal situation. How could something be constant across all of humanity and yet not have a biological basis?

If the unconscious were purely relational, its structures (Id, Ego, Superego, Preconscious, etc.) would vary significantly in their existence and functions from individual to individual and group to group. There would be no singular translational activity or consistent function—there might be billions of variations, but this is not the case. Laplanche asserts that translational activity is present within the Fundamental Anthropological Situation, and he speaks of moments when it is activated, implying that it must already exist. To the best of my knowledge, he never uses the term "created." Instead, he uses terms like "activated" or "stimulated," which imply something pre-existing rather than newly formed. I believe it aligns entirely with Laplanche's thinking to acknowledge that something may have a biological origin, as most aspects of our lives do, but then undergoes transformation—and this is where the concept of emergent properties becomes significant.

I believe Laplanche conceptualizes the Fundamental Situation as one in which sexual message is implanted in the child's body, and this is universal. It may occur as implantation in its ordinary form, or as intromission when the message becomes intrusive and potentially superegoic, but it is always present. Without contact with the sexuality of the other, one cannot become fully "human." To develop this humanity, contact with others is essential, and for Laplanche, this contact is inherently with the sexual other. The other implants a stimulus within you, which arouses your body, and Laplanche suggests that there is likely a receptor in the body prepared to receive it. If it is implanted in the body, it is because the body is inherently ready to receive it.

BBT: As you know, Laplanche developed the compromised message after he abandoned the concept of leaning-on, but it's almost like you're situating leaning-on and the compromised message on a continuum. Could you say little bit more about that?

JCC: "Leaning-on" refers to our instinctual tendencies for self-preservation and species survival from birth. Seeking out the mother is part of this attachment, a fundamental survival mechanism that makes us receptive to both the mother's presence and her messages. Unlike other animals that are born with more developed structures, many of which can walk, find food, or regulate their body temperature—humans are born extremely helpless. This dependence means we must establish a connection with others, particularly the mother, for survival. I believe this unique need for contact has been shaped through evolution.

BBT: That would be the aspect of leaning-on, the peeling off.

JCC: We are born with an *embodied dependency* on another for our survival. It's not ontologically about desiring love; it's about the need to survive. We instinctively connect to another member of our species, forming an attachment to whoever is caring for us. My perspective, drawing on Laplanche's ideas, is that in this state of attachment, we are open to countless messages from the other because we need to communicate—to send and receive messages. Then comes a completely different kind of message, unrelated to survival: the sexually charged message. This message is not natural in the sense of being instinctual, as our sexuality is not driven by reproductive instincts. Instead, our sexual interests are linked to satisfying desires, to engaging with partial objects, and to our fantasies of infantile sexuality. There are no natural codes at play here. While we use our instincts for the physical act of sexual intercourse, our desires and wishes to relate sexually to others arise from our fantasies—rooted in infantile sexuality. When this sexual message arrives, and we engage our translational function to process it, we create something new, by evolutionary chance. Through this translational activity, we produce meaning, though this is not due to any teleological intention.

We produce meaning because it is in our nature to do so after the activity of translation—each of our emotional experiences gains meaning through this process. The only way meaning is not produced is if one is in a part of the mental structure that is not psychic or if translational activity has not been activated—in the *enclaved* unconscious, everything remains untranslated. Laplanche makes this clear: Untranslated messages do not produce meaning. Meaning arises after the creation of the preconscious, which itself is formed through translational activity. Laplanche frequently emphasizes that translational activity is what generates all psychic spaces. How could it create the same psychic spaces in every individual since the beginning of humanity if it were not a constant force? If it is indeed constant—an invariant—throughout human evolution, it must be biological. There is no other known plausible explanation.

Regarding the emergent property, it is what Laplanche refers to as "emergence"; in English, we may use either "emergent property" or "emergence." This emergent property is what truly defines our humanity. Our humanity arises from having a conscious/unconscious structure, psychic spaces, and fundamentally, the ability to attribute meaning to our emotional experiences. The unconscious is formed through translational activity and the production of meaning. All of the preconscious is about meaning, and the sexuality that persists there after translation will create the unconscious through repression. Some messages are so dominated by sexuality that they are sent back to the *enclaved* unconscious.

Previously, you asked whether this was extending beyond the boundaries of psychoanalysis. It is not. On the contrary, it provides a crucial perspective for understanding psychoanalysis in relation to the disciplines we recognize today, rather than turning it into something incomprehensible—often dismissed as "magical thinking" or pseudoscience, as Popper suggested. I do not believe psychoanalysis is pseudoscience; it has its own epistemology, rooted in immateriality and the complex relationship with the other and others. However, analysts tend to resist engaging with biology. Psychoanalysts often find it easier to connect with sociology than with biology, which I see as a limitation.

BBT: That reminds me of something that came up earlier. You said when you were an editor of *The International Journal of Psychoanalysis* that you recognized how important epistemology is relative to culture, and I think that keeps coming up in relation to a lot of what we're talking about today because there's a massive differentiation between epistemology and culture. My question is, how would you characterize epistemology as a method of psychoanalytic research and practice? What is the relationship between Laplanche's epistemology and culture, which is to say, is there a way of not being swept up by the mytho-symbolic and thus going astray?

JCC: First, it's essential to define what we mean when discussing epistemology. I don't see it as a method in itself but rather as a structure in our thinking. In the context of psychoanalytic research and practice, you are not conducting epistemological research directly; instead, epistemology serves as a foundational framework for reflection. It prompts questions like: What exactly are we trying to understand here? How does this relate to other disciplines? What is the underlying structure of this thought? What is the origin of this concept? What are the conditions for a specific justified belief?

For instance, I believe it's essential to emphasize that Laplanche focuses on stimulating translational activity in the session through the concept of "*refusement*." Although "*refusement*" is not a proper English term, it conveys the idea more accurately than "refusal" and is closer to the original French meaning. To fully grasp this concept, it's crucial to understand the underlying meaning and context of what he is expressing.

Expanding on this example, Bion suggests that you must listen to the patient without desire, memory, or the intention to cure. To understand what Bion intended, it's essential to recognize that he sought a new emotional experience in each session. He aimed to develop a method that would allow him to connect with what was emotionally new in the communication. When people dismiss Bion's method as impractical, arguing that one cannot work without memory, desire, or the wish to cure, they fail to grasp what he was striving for. When Laplanche discusses *refusement*, he aims to stimulate the process of generating meaning. This *refusement* is intended to promote the re-establishment of the Fundamental Anthropological Situation within the session.

In my view, *refusement* is a crucial part of re-establishing the stimulation of translational activity within the session. In a way, when Bion speaks of trying to be without memory and desire in order to engage with the new, I interpret it as implying that one must adopt a position of *refusement* to connect with the Fundamental Anthropological Situation and activate the capacity to create symbols and meaning. I believe this lies at the heart of Laplanche's ideas and is central to working with hollowed-out transference. These issues are part of epistemological inquiry—a theory of knowledge.

BBT: There's an argument made that because of *après-coup* and the temporality of *après-coup*, later in time, someone might realize that they were misgendered, and they're a man, or a woman, or nonbinary, and that changes with time. There's an ongoing experience of being as compared to an ontological "I am." This way, there's an ongoing experience of being that's rewritten through the temporality of *après-coup*. How do you see that concept? Is that an ideology? Is that a misreading of Laplanche? How would you think about that?

JCC: I agree that *après-coup* alters meaning. Changing meaning inevitably transforms the self—there is an evolution that takes place. However, everything we are discussing is emotional and unconscious, with a level of complexity that is perhaps the most profound we encounter. Not even quantum physics matches this intricacy. The number of interactions and variables involved is immense and highly complex, necessitating a deeply abstract model of representation. It is not at all conscious, so there is no possibility of imagining this as a deliberate choice in a given moment. You may realize that something was flawed in your constitution—that something that should have been integrated was not. You come to this realization, and if you are in contact with your unconscious, you are able to work it through with great effort and integrate it differently. But this process is neither cognitive nor conscious in any way.

BBT: You said that *après-coup* functions as a temporality that's unconscious. Could you just flesh that out a little bit more? What do you mean by that?

JCC: I'm not sure I fully understand your question, but there are four dimensions of temporality. The dimension we are discussing—the *après-coup* dimension—is a movement of the unconscious. It involves creating a new meaning of the sexual message where there was none before or where there was a different meaning, and this process is driven by the translation of the messages. The movement of *après-coup* draws its energy from the act of translation. Everything we are discussing here is unconscious; it's not about consciously thinking differently. While you can do that, it remains within the realm of the conscious. In addition to this, there are cognitive thinking, cultural influences, and many other factors, but these are not what *après-coup* refers to.

BBT: What are the other dimensions of temporality? You said there were four.

JCC: In the article "Temporalité et Traduction" (2008), Laplanche makes reference to four temporalities that originate from philosophical studies, encompassing views from philosophy, physics, and psychology. Laplanche's aim is to introduce a philosophy of time into psychoanalysis, based on the concept of *après-coup*.

Throughout this chapter, Laplanche engages in profound reflections on the distinction between time and temporality, emphasizing that the notion of temporality is separated from the conventional notion of time by introducing a necessary personal experience of time as lived by the individual.

A concise overview of the commonly referenced notions of time includes:

1 **Linear Time (Chronos)**. This is the conventional, conscious understanding and experience of time—progressing linearly from past to present to future. It is how we measure events in our lives and arrange them in a logical sequence. Linear time is often used in cognitive processes and planning, encompassing the idea of a "starting point" and an "ending."
2 **Circular or Cyclical Time** is characterized by the repetition of cycles, such as days, seasons, or natural biological rhythms. This understanding of time

is common in many traditional cultures and reflects natural processes, like the changing of seasons, the cycle of birth and death, and the recurrence of experiences that follow a familiar pattern. In contemporary development and philosophy of mind literature, the rhythms of the mother-infant relationship are also described as fundamental components for emotional regulation, the development of secure attachment, and the influence on cognitive and sensorimotor growth, including the establishment of intersubjectivity. Laplanche, in the mentioned chapter, links these rhythms to pleasure-unpleasure experiences.

3 **Kairos** (sometimes referred to as opportune or authentic time) represents qualitative time, focusing on the opportune moment when something significant can happen. Kairos refers to time as an experience rather than a measurable entity, suggesting a critical point when action, transformation, or decision making is most effective.

Après-coup does not follow a specific pace. It represents a change in meaning due to a transformation, reflecting a different concept of temporality.

The English translations, "afterwardsness" or "deferred action," do not precisely capture the sense of movement. According to Laplanche, we begin with a message that must hold meaning. It must have meaning because it generates an economic disequilibrium within, as the presence of sexuality creates excitement. This is the starting point and reveals the necessity of translation. It produces an economic disequilibrium—as Freud described with the economic principle, and as Laplanche reiterated in many of his texts—which lies at the core of the issue. Excitation is at the heart of the problem, and it must be transformed (or bound).

My idea is that evolution provides us with a solution, which is translation—the creation of meaning. In the process of creating meaning, we first bind elements. Binding is fundamental here, as it allows us to manage the element of excitation, which, when unbound, represents the *sexual* death drive. When bound, it represents the *sexual* life drive. Excitation lies at the center, and it can either be bound or left unbound. Translation must bind and provide a sense of ownership; it belongs to you rather than being something alien within you. Through translation, we form a meaning that feels personally ours. Although we produce meanings influenced by the mytho-symbolic, they are ultimately individual. This is why we are singular beings rather than part of an undifferentiated mass.

Laplanche emphasizes several times that translation occurs in two phases: the moment of receiving the message and the moment of translating it. When we receive the message, it lacks meaning. The message carries an implicit meaning, but no one knows what it is—neither the recipient nor the sender—because it originates from the unconscious of the sender, making it impossible to know. Then, we create a meaning, and this process is dynamic. It involves transformation and even displacement, moving from the *enclaved* unconscious to the preconscious and then into the repressed unconscious. This movement is central to Laplanche's thinking, with *après-coup* at its core, as it is a process that repeats, given that the message can only ever be partially translated.

Some messages are impossible to translate because their sexual content is excessive (for example, Calich, 2006). Laplanche refers to these as hypersexualized messages (Laplanche, 2006). In such cases, translation is not possible, and the messages remain exciting, retaining their sexual nature and waiting for a retrospective attempt of translation.

If a message can be translated, another movement takes place: sublimation, through which we produce a new meaning, *après-coup*. This process requires ongoing translation, promoting an expansion of the psychic world and enabling the possibility of constituting and integrating ourselves into culture and relationships with others. This movement is sublimation and, along with its temporality, is the essence of *après-coup*.

Notes

1 A more in-depth elaboration of the concept of *refusement* appears in Chapter 3.
2 "Il reste que, si l'analyse se propose de défaire ces traductions imparfaites que lui présente le patient: sa vie actuelle, ses rêves, ses symptômes, il faut bien qu'il existe déjà, dans l'existence humaine en général, quelque chose que soi un mouvement de traduction et de détraduction-retraduction."
3 In Chapter 4, there is a further explication of the complementary and similar aspects of Laplanche's and Aulagnier's theories.

Bibliography

Calich, J. C. (2006). Pour "faire travailler" la topique laplanchienne. *Psychiatrie française, 37*(3), 34–44.

Calich, J. C. (2021). Comentário ao texto *Acerca da minha concepção do Eu,* de Jean Laplanche [Commentary on the text "About my conception of the Ego," by Jean Laplanche]. *Revista de Psicanálise da SPPA, 28*(3).

Freud, S. (2016). *Three essays on the theory of sexuality: The 1905 edition* (U. Kistner, Trans.). Verso.

Laplanche, J. (2006). Reponse à José Carlos Calich. Le concept d'inconscient selon Jean Laplanche. *Psychiatrie française, 37*(3), 44–46.

Laplanche, J. (2008). *La révolution copernicienne inachevée. 1967–1992*. PUF.

Laplanche, J. (2011). *Freud and the sexual.* The Unconscious in Translation.

Laplanche, J. (2015). *Problématiques V: Le baquet. Transcendance du transfert*. PUF.

Laplanche, J. (2021). *Acerca da minha concepção do Eu* [About my conception of the Ego]. *Revista de Psicanálise da SPPA, 28*(3).

Laplanche, J., & Fletcher, J. (2005). *Essays on otherness*. Routledge.

Laplanche, J., & House, J. (2016). *New foundations for psychoanalysis*. The Unconscious in Translation.

Laplanche, J., House, J., & Thurston, L. (2017). *Après-coup: Problématiques VI*. The Unconscious in Translation.

Laplanche, J., & Mehlman, J. (2015). *Between seduction and inspiration: Man*. The Unconscious in Translation.

Laplanche, J., & Thurston, L. (2020). *The unfinished Copernican revolution: Selected works, 1967–1992*. The Unconscious in Translation.

Martens, F. (2006). Le concept d'inconscient selon Jean Laplanche. *Psychiatrie française, 37*(3), 131–135.

Tarelho, L. C. (2021). Apresentação do texto *Acerca da minha concepção do Eu*, de Jean Laplanche [Presentation of the text "About my conception of the Ego," by Jean Laplanche]. *Revista de Psicanálise da SPPA, 28*(3).

7 Isabelle Gernet

Université Paris Cité, Paris, France

Translated from the French into English.

Bryan Batista-Thomas: Could you tell me a little bit about how you came to Laplanche's work?

Isabelle Gernet: My encounter with Laplanche's work originated in my psychology thesis, which looked at the psychological changes caused by epilepsy neurosurgery. While the severe epileptic seizures from which the patients suffered ceased with the surgical procedure, the patients developed psychopathological decompensation. The elucidation of these psychosomatic problems led me to take an interest in the role of the other in neurosurgical care, with the main hypothesis being that the care work carried out by the caregivers is an opportunity to revive the dynamics of original seduction and the impasses of seduction through mobilizing the patient's erotic body.

In rejecting the psyche/soma dichotomy, Laplanche maintains a reservation about the status of the body and its experiences in both the genesis of psychic life and the dynamics of sublimation, which is tested in the psychosomatic clinic. My own research, based on my clinical experience with patients presenting with somatic pathologies, as well as psychopathological decompensations linked to work, seeks to show how the General Theory of Seduction emerges as an original theory capable of accounting for the place of the body, on the one hand, and of society, on the other, in the genesis of psychic reality.

The model of the General Theory of Seduction is in fact a metapsychological theory of the links between subject and society, which is not directly inscribed in psychic reality, but instead operates through the compromised messages of adults implanted in the child's body.

On the basis of Laplanche's critique of representation, some of the metapsychological issues involved in analytic practice with patients suffering in ways that specifically concern the question of the body in psychosomatics,

DOI: 10.4324/9781032670287-8

on the one hand, and its relationship to work, on the other, are based on the impasses of sublimation.

In truth, these two paths are closely articulated around the metapsychology of the message and the impasses of seduction sedimenting in the form of an entrenched unconscious.

BBT: When you speak about metapsychology, are you referring to metapsychology of representation or metapsychology of the message?

IG: The theoretical and practical questions raised by the psychosomatic clinic have helped to expand the debate between psychoanalytic practitioners on the boundaries between what can be analyzed and what is "unrepresented." In Freud's work, the concept of representation is closely linked to a theory of perception. From the "Project for a Scientific Psychology" onwards, a dialectical model emerges between the construction of an "ego" in opposition to the external world, which makes itself known through perceptions.

The Freudian theory of psychic work, conceived as the specific work of representation, is presented as the result of the conflicting destinies of the dialectic of external perceptions (as received by the perception-consciousness system) and internal perceptions (the drives). The primacy accorded to representation was accompanied by the growing importance given by Freud to external reality, which culminated in his reflections on splitting and the capacity of the ego to "fissure," or divide, as a result of confrontation with external constraints.

For Freud, the model of perception underlying the differentiation between inside and outside explains the genesis of psychic life based on a metapsychological conception of the mnesic trace. The constitution of the first traces is thus linked to original repression, the origin of the traces connecting them to the hallucinatory realization and the experience of what Freud designates as "satisfaction" and the meaning given to it. The metapsychological model of "hallucination" as a specific activity of psychic life refers primarily to the concept of the absent object and the subjective capacity to bring it into existence (in other words, to hallucinate it) in its absence, as a condition of subjective life.

Metapsychological conceptions of the memory trace suggest that the representation, as the residue of perception, is always the mark of an external object, thereby introducing confusion between what Laplanche calls "psychological reality," made up of memories and perceptual remains, and what would constitute "psychic reality." Based on the Fundamental Anthropological Situation, which is characterized by an asymmetrical relationship between adult and child, the General Theory of Seduction, on the other hand, emphasizes the role played by the enigmatic nature of the adult's compromised sexual messages to the child. From the point of view of the General Theory of Seduction, psychic reality is not reduced to a subjective reality conceived according to the model of hallucinatory satisfaction but is established as radically foreign, because the message implanted by the adult in the child's body is de-qualified.

For Laplanche, the message conveys not a latent content—related to the adult's fantasies—but a traumatic excitation that the child will have to translate. Let us recall here the conceptual differences between Freud's concept of arousal and Laplanche's use of the term (Gernet, 2020). For Laplanche, the term "arousal" refers specifically to sexual arousal, which enables him to underline the ambiguities of Freud's use of the term "arousal" and its "biologizing" purpose.

The implanted message at the core of the drive is "de-signified," meaning that the original repression initiated by the first translations is not based on a process of representation starting from the perceptual traces of the object. This, moreover, leads Laplanche to reject the classical opposition between the representation of a thing and the representation of a word. The reference to representation is supplanted by the category of message.

The core of the unconscious is thus made up of "thing-representations" conceived, not as perceptual remains, but as "what escapes the child's first attempts to construct an interhuman world" (Laplanche, 1987, p. 80). This conception allows Laplanche to abandon the dualism of "pure factuality and creative imagination" (Laplanche, 1991, p. 409) and situate the origin of psychic life in interhuman communication rather than in biological life. The reference to the message is presented as constituting a reality of its own, "a third order of reality, not alongside material reality and psychological reality, but transversal to them: the reality of the message, the materiality of which must be called the 'signifier'" (Laplanche, 1999, p. 131). The essence of the sexual and of psychic reality can thus be characterized in relation to the dimension of the exciting enigma of the message to be translated.

BBT: The metapsychology of the message?

IG: Yes, to continue along the path of the metapsychology of the message is to move towards a paradigm that displaces the represented/unrepresented pair—a classic opposition, particularly in the field of psychoanalytic psychosomatics—towards that of the *translated/untranslatable*.

Whereas partial failures of translation account for the formation of the repressed sexual unconscious at the root of the neurotic-normal mode of psychic functioning, *radical failures of translation* organize the constitution of the unconscious designated as "embedded" or "subconscious" because none of the message could be translated. In the case of radical failures of translation, Laplanche insists on the persistence of the message in its primary form within the psychic apparatus: "the original message remains as it is in the psychic apparatus, implanted or intromitted."

For Laplanche, clinical situations linked to the radical failure of translation present themselves as a major practical problem for analysts faced with cases that deviate from the neurotic-normal model, which is one of the psychopathological discussion points for patients presenting serious somatic pathologies. Without translation, the forming of the preconscious, which "corresponds to the way in which the subject constitutes himself and represents his history" (2003b, p. 218), is hindered, leading to the *enclaved* unconscious—in Laplanche's conception—"flush with consciousness," that is, in direct contact with reality in an "apparently logical and 'operative' mode" (2003b, p. 218).

These clinical situations, analyzed in the light of the untranslatable and the embedded unconscious, pose new practical problems, insofar as the "aim of the analytical process" in this case would not be to move from the unrepresented to a representation, but rather to encourage the resumption of the work of translation on the basis of the emergence of new registers of experience involving the body. The General Theory of Seduction thus makes it possible to revisit the conditions of "psychic treatment" (Freud) of the bodily states that psychosomatic theorizations have revealed, by moving away from the model of hysterical conversion proposed by Freud.

BBT: Could you expand on the metapsychology of the message and its relationship to sublimation?

IG: Although the sublimatory value of ordinary work [referring to jobs and a career] is far from being recognized in the psychoanalytical field, we can nevertheless demonstrate, with the backing of clinical evidence, that work mobilizes *all* of subjectivity. The gestures performed at work can be harnessed for symbolization, because they mobilize the body to construct meaning. The specific constraints of the work situation (physical as well as social constraints) can thus take on the value of a message and trigger the need for psychic work.

The specific constraints of work (not only physical but also social constraints) may be understood as a message, thus triggering the need for psychic work regarding the mode of translation/de-translation/re-translation of childhood enigmatic messages. This work of (re)interpretation is based on the elaboration of psycho-emotional and sublimatory impasses that are revived in the subjective relation to work. Exercising an occupation and acquiring "professional" experience demand an important mobilization of psychic life, which Freud himself only partially described in *Civilization and Its Discontents* (1929): "It is not possible to discuss the significance of work for the economics of the libido adequately within the limits of a short survey. Laying stress upon importance of work has a greater effect than any other technique of living in the direction of binding the individual more closely to reality; in his work he is at least securely attached to a part of reality, the human community" (Freud, p. 34).

The psychic resources of the subjective mobilization of individuals to resolve the difficulties stemming from work-related constraints draw on epistemophilia and the source-object of the drives related to the enigmatic messages of childhood. These enigmatic messages, as sources of excitement to be translated, are closely intertwined with translation work required when encountering resistance from the material reality of the work situation, a situation that is always structured by physical and technical constraints, not to mention social constraints. By reaffirming the primacy of sexuality in the psychic dynamic, Laplanche's theory defends an original conception of psychic life that does not overlook the social relations of domination.

For Laplanche, the Fundamental Anthropological Situation (based on the General Theory of Seduction) is a fundamental fact of human nature in which the child unavoidably experiences inequality in relationships, which stems from the problem of assignment. His theory on gender assignment is linked to the identification of the baby's gender *by* the adults. Laplanche regards this as the "primacy of the other" in the assignment process: Here, the child does not *identify himself or herself as* but is rather *identified by* (Laplanche, 2007), thus stressing the enigmatic aspect of any gender assignment by adults, which is inevitably compromised by the child's own sexual unconscious. In analytic practice with patients who present diverse forms of work-related suffering, a process is initiated to redefine the notion of assignment not only from the perspective of gender assignment but also as a theoretical link to explain the conflictual relation between sexuality and the social sphere. This redefinition leads to a conception that radically differs from the theories of the intersubjectivist tradition on the genesis of psychic processes (cf. H. Tessier, 2007).

BBT: How is this represented in the clinic?

IG: In psychoanalysis and clinical psychopathology, the majority of observations formally state: "[T]his is a man in his thirties, a woman in her twenties, an analyst, etc..." *whose work consists of* ... we might add. The experience of work, by inscribing the subject in social relations, reiterates the enigma of the origin of the subject. In other words, work presents itself as a non-"ipso-centric" experience, the main characteristic of which is to take into account "the child in the presence of the adult and receiving from her/him messages that are not raw data, but that need 'to be translated'" (Laplanche 2003a, p. 180), which contributes to relaunching the subject's work of self-theorization.

The Laplanchean model thus makes it possible to revisit the traditional relationships between inside and outside, between psychic reality and material reality on the basis of the category of message. From this perspective, social reproduction (as in the case of gender, but also more broadly in the case of social domination) is not "internalized" by the psyche but is submitted to the subject's work of translation. The codes and narrative schemas that Laplanche sees as constituting the category of the mytho-symbolic (or pseudo-unconscious) play a part in the process of historicization of the subject and serve to bind the sexual together through translation.

BBT: As you mentioned previously, there is a difference between the neurotic individual and the person in the psychosomatic clinic; can you speak a little about the latter's presentation?

IG: While the psychosomatic clinic is organized around an "operative" mode of functioning that leaves little room for association-based thinking, the clinic of work also reveals the disorders that affect the thought process. In the patient's discourse, we find thought content and forms of "borrowed" discourse based on stereotypes and conformism, which can be seen as "resistance" mobilized by the analysand in the context of the analytical work. When the subject embarks on the path of translating enigmatic messages and repeating them iteratively on the basis of confrontation with social constraints, the translation process relies in part on the translation aids provided by myths as "instruments for putting things into narrative."

However, Laplanche points out, with regard to the narrative structures, codes, and myths proposed by the social world, that "the 'knowledge' value of these codes is non-existent, whereas their potential for linking and shaping is undeniable. They belong to the realm of ideology" (Laplanche, 1998, p. 250). The General Theory of Seduction reveals the ambiguity of the ego in charge of connection, always confronted with the risk of immobilization through imaginary synthesis (by gestalt). Hence Laplanche's constant preoccupation with analyzing the issue of translation and, in particular, sublimation as an "open" mode of symbolization.

In "Sublimation and/or Inspiration," in *Between Seduction and Inspiration: Man*, Laplanche reintroduced the distinction between different types of connection by identifying the narcissistic connection, which is said to serve phallic narcissism and defenses, as opposed to the symbolic connection made up of translation/de-translation/re-translation. Both are considered to be at the service of the ego, which raises the paradox of an ego oriented toward growth through the process of acculturation and the transposition of death drives into life drives, on the one hand, and likely to be captured by "crude" narcissistic connections, on the other. This paradox also concerns sublimation and its risk of "Ptolemaic" closure: "I don't see how we can distinguish this progression of Eros, in each individual existence—mainly by means of symbolization—from sublimation. It is sublimation itself, as the integration of anarchic sexual goals into a 'socially valued' perspective" (Laplanche, 1999, p. 323).

BBT: You raised the notion of gestalt or narcissistic binding in comparison to the more nuanced symbolic binding. Could you speak to its place in the psychosomatic clinic given the different mode of functioning?

IG: This theoretical work of discussion with Laplanche's theses is still in progress, in particular through the search for the origin of Laplanche's use of the term "gestalt" to designate the constitution of a specific form

> of connection by the ego in an imaginary relationship. The search for "forms" designated by the term "gestalt" evokes what philosopher Ernst Cassirer would have sought to characterize by the expression "symbolic pervasiveness." The identification of "levels of symbolization," depending on the nature of the connection, can be put to the test in clinical situations that confront the clinician with impasses or obstacles to the thinking process.

In work-related psychopathology, the clinic of the defenses against suffering reveals the psychic processes involved in the subjects' ability to temporarily stop themselves from thinking. The suffering caused by difficulties in the workplace is countered by defenses, which, in some cases, significantly impact the ability to think and to elaborate the subjective relation to work constraints. These defenses, despite their utility in permitting the continuation of work, lead to a marked decline in spontaneous thought while creating the economy of anxiety.

Affecting the thinking of workers, these disorders can paradoxically play an important role in the subjective resources of consent and servitude to domination, which perpetuate the suffering (Dejours, 2006). Most defensive constructions rely on the partial denial of perception and rationalization, fueled by the psychological investment of ideological content transmitted by the social imagination. The ideological system involved in many modes of defense against work-related suffering is based on social virility, which is particularly effective at keeping the unconscious offshoots linked to the experience of suffering outside the realm of thought by overinvesting the conscious system.

Indeed, social virility, by rewarding the social attributes associated with men and the masculine, such as performance, courage, strength, power, and mastery, accords privileges in social relations associated with the domination of those who cannot be virile. The overinvestment of the conscious system thus leads to a bipartite division of psychic life by erecting a separation between the different areas of life (split between personal life and professional life) and/or forms of thought (associative thought versus conformist or even "operational" thought). In the case of work-related psychopathological decompensation, the preservation of this "double blind" situation, which can sometimes remain functional throughout the entire lifetime, is disrupted and often plunged into a serious crisis. This clinic of work allows me to apply Laplanche's propositions regarding the formation of a split unconscious, which designates a topographical system—distinct from the repressed sexual unconscious—formed by untranslated messages that result from the radical failures of translation but also by the compromised messages yet to be translated.

For Laplanche, the failures of translation, which are responsible for the impasses in symbolization, lie in the gap between implantation and intromission, arising from the status accorded to the code as a "translation aid," paving the way for the process of semiotization/translation. In the case of implantation, the intrusion by the message of the other and the search for translation that it gives rise to are at the root of the simultaneous constitution of the sexual unconscious and the ego, as the capacity to measure oneself on the basis of the task of thinking. In the case of intromission, the impossibility of translating the message seems to be at the root of the constitution of psychic *enclaves* formed by proscription, at the root of profound alterations in the work of thinking.

Recourse to a crude mode of linking the ego, as a tendency of psychic life, would thus be "actualized" in certain social situations, which Laplanche suggests are related to the development of specific social relationships: "[O]ne cannot fail to notice that with abstract and generalized exchanges a kind of regression occurs from the partial object to the index, from the life drive to the death drive, and with it, a desublimation. It must be said, moreover, that the partial object, by virtue of being partial, already conceals a meaning of weapon and deadly projectile, which Melanie Klein never ceased to emphasize." In an article dating from 1921, Marcel Mauss already emphasized the two meanings of the Germanic word "gift": gift and poison: "the thing received (…) coming from one, made or appropriated by him, being of him, confers power over the other who accepts it" (Laplanche, 1999, p. 321).

Bibliography

Dejours, C. (2006). Subjectivity, work, and action. *Critical Horizons, 7*(1), 45–62. https://doi.org/10.1163/156851606779308161

Freud, S. (1915). Repression. In J. Strachey (Ed. & Trans.), *The standard edition of the complete psychological works of Sigmund Freud* (Vol. 14, pp. 141–158). Hogarth Press.

Freud, S. (1930). Civilization and its discontents. In J. Strachey (Ed. & Trans.), SE (Vol. 21, pp. 57–146). Hogarth Press.

Freud, S. (1950). Project for a scientific psychology (1895). In J. Strachey (Ed. & Trans.), SE (Vol. 1, pp. 281–391). Hogarth Press.

Gernet, I. (2020). Théorie de la séduction généralisée et théorie du sens: À propos des obstacles au travail de penser. In H. Tessier (Ed.), *Psychanalyse et théorie du sens: Un dialogue entre la pensée de Jean Laplanche et la sémiotique* (pp. 189–218). PUF. https://doi.org/10.3917/puf.tessi.2021.01.0189

Laplanche, J. (1987). *Nouveaux fondements pour la psychanalyse*. PUF.

Laplanche, J. (1991), *Le primat de l'autre en psychanalyse*. Flammarion.

Laplanche, J. (1999). *Entre séduction et inspiration: L'homme*. PUF.

Laplanche, J. (2003a). Gender, sex, and the *sexual*. In *Freud and the sexual: Essays, 2000–2006* (pp. 167–209). The Unconscious in Translation.

Laplanche, J. (2003b). Three meanings of the term 'Unconscious' in the framework of the general theory of seduction. In *Freud and the sexual: Essays, 2000–2006* (pp. 190–245). The Unconscious in Translation.

Laplanche, J. (2007). *Sexual: La sexualité élargie au sens freudien*. PUF.

Laplanche, J. (2008). *La révolution copernicienne inachevée. 1967–1992*. PUF.
Mauss, M. (1954). *The gift: Forms and functions of exchange in archaic societies* (I. Cunnison, Trans.). Cohen & West.
Tessier, H. (2007). Pulsion et subjectivité. *Libres cahiers pour la psychanalyse, 15*(1), 129–147. https://doi.org/10.3917/lcpp.015.0129

8 Nicolas Evzonas

Université Paris Cité, Institut de l'Association psychanalytique de France, Paris, France

Bryan Batista-Thomas: We were discussing the methodological part of translation and the word "translation" in German, meaning both transference and translation. Going further, we covered the way in which Laplanche was positioned as being an actual translator and having perhaps a transference to the text. However, I believe Lacan was often saying he had, and that one needs to have a transference to Freud and to the text. Laplanche was very much against that. There is a book, I am sure you know it, about Laplanche and translation.

Nicolas Evzonas: Yes, it's *Traduire Freud [Translating Freud]*, but I was not referring to this one, although it's very useful. Since I work with the French texts, in *Essays on Otherness*, the English translation of the edited volume *The Unfinished Copernican Revolution*, refers to the de-centeredness and otherness. I think that the English title—*Essays on Otherness*—translates in a free way the content of the book. There are maybe four or five essays in this book where Laplanche speaks about the translation of Freud's work.

What was really striking for me was to read Laplanche's guidelines about the translation he was doing at the time. Laplanche was the scientific director of the committee translating the complete works by Freud from German into French. Laplanche described his methodological principles of interlinguistic translation in different papers than those in which he elaborated the metapsychological translational model. It is perhaps not surprising that someone who devoted himself to the translation of Freud's complete work viewed clinical practice and thus the emergence of psychic life in light of the notion of translation. This "coincidence" would appear to be supported by the German language, like the noun *Übersetzung*, which means both translation and transference. We may consider that translation in the "restricted sense" (i.e., interlinguistic translation)

DOI: 10.4324/9781032670287-9

and translation in the "extended sense" (i.e., metapsychological translational model) constitute two dimensions of the same problem. The most striking common feature of these two seemingly different practices is the primacy of the other.

Freud, translator of Charcot and Stuart Mill, recommended reading an entire page or passage from the original, then closing the book and writing, asking oneself: "How can this be rendered in German?". Contrastingly, Laplanche translated by prioritizing not the target language – French _but the source language – German –, hence the language of the other. Regarding his metapsychological translational model, Laplanche postulates that sexuality and psychic life arise under the aegis of the primordial others and their enigmatic signifiers. If we take into consideration Laplanche's interlinguistic translation and metapsychological translational model, we can argue that the groundbreaking theory bequeathed to us by Laplanche is less of a "general seduction" (the official name of his theory) than a "generalized translation."

In the essay "Transference: Its Provocation by the Analyst," Laplanche clearly speaks about the transference outside the clinical setting and about the transference onto culture and the messages that we receive from society. However, what I'm trying to say is that Laplanche has this broader idea of transference. A transference that goes far beyond the clinical setting. Indeed, transference and countertransference are not just clinical notions.

You were telling me earlier that you had difficulty listening to patients and having several psychoanalytic theories in mind, which seemed very limited or normative. What you were saying, I think as well, was about your transference to these theories. In my view, countertransference does not only include the revival of infantile desires and anxieties in the analyst's psyche. It also entails the introjection of technical, methodological, and psychopathological references which shape the analyst's listening. For me, theoretical countertransference determines clinical countertransference.

I'm translating in my own words what I got from you when you were speaking with me about how all these theories about sexuality didn't speak to you. They didn't make any sense, whereas the Laplanchean framework allows you to listen to your patients without normalizing them. I can totally understand that, because our multiple transferences toward theories, supervisors, psychoanalytic societies, theoretical fathers and mothers shape our listening. Laplanche has also helped me to broaden my listening because his theories are free from any normativity.

There are so many references in Laplanche to Freud, Ferenczi, and Margaret Mead. Let me first recall that Laplanche doesn't speak about family, parents and children. Following Ferenczi, he refers to adults in a position of authority. What really concerns Laplanche is the anthropological asymmetry between adults and the child, and this is an influence by Ferenczi. The latter was the first to speak about the *adult's* language and the intrinsically different *child's* language. Both Ferenczi and Laplanche emancipate psychoanalysis from its familistic perspective, which was rightfully criticized by Gilles Deleuze, Felix Guattari, and Michel Foucault. It is also interesting to remember that Laplanche, in *Nouveaux Fondements de psychanalyse*, explicitly mentions Ferenczi, thus saying that the confusion of tongues paradigm constitutes the preface of his own theory of generalized seduction.

Laplanche further quotes the work of Margaret Mead, and argues that the fact that a child is reared by his/her/their parents is a cultural and social contingency. We do have other kinds of relatedness, which do not abide by family structures. But what we have as an anthropological invariant, which doesn't change no matter what culture or society, is this Fundamental Anthropological Situation: Which is this asymmetry between the adults and the child. Aside from the emancipation of psychoanalysis from familial imperialism through the introduction of the anthropological dyad adults/child, Laplanche further de-genders the primary objects. As mentioned earlier, he doesn't speak about a mother or a father, he speaks about adults who send enigmatic messages to the child.

In his 2003 essay "Gender, Sex, and the *Sexual*," he proposes the notion of the *socius proche*. This can be translated as the intimate *socius*. By this term, Laplanche means the primordial others during childhood, that is, caregivers, and a constellation of libidinally invested adults. What is important for me is that Laplanche pluralizes the objects and identificatory figures, as well as the messages which circulate between adults and the child. Laplanche does not remain ensnared in the traditional nuclear family triangle. He speaks about multiple enigmatic messages from many senders with ongoing translations. Hence, an endless reshaping of subjectivity. I consider Laplanche as a precursor of queer studies because he pluralizes primary objects, messages, translations, while de-gendering caregivers, which is even more relevant today given the new sociological configurations of homosexual parenting and trans parenting, as well as surrogate mothers and sperm donors who add complexity and plurality to the child's fantasmatic world.

BBT: I did a word check to see if I could find the exact translation for *socius proche*.

NE: Thomas Burkhalter, a Laplanchean scholar from South Africa translates this as "intimate *socius*."[1]

BBT: John Fletcher seems to have translated it as "*socius*." There's no specification.

NE: Well, we should think of the context where Laplanche uses the term *socius*: he actually writes that gender is not assigned by society in general, but by the intimate *socius*. He could have said by the people from the intimate circle of the child, but I think that he uses the word *socius* to suggest that the adults around the child are socially inserted and consequently they are purveyors of the social. From a Laplanchean perspective, social and cultural norms are transmitted to the child by caregivers and other people from the intimate *socius* who are already inscribed into the social. That said, norms are not directly transmitted to the child. Instead, they're transmitted as enigmatic messages to be translated by the child. In other words, norms are transmitted through the mediation of the adults' unconscious and are assimilated by the child according to his or her own idiosyncratic translational abilities.

BBT: I'm curious, given that we're talking about translations, there are some things that I have found that have been translated from French into English in such a way that meaning is changed. For example, *indice* is used in French but not in English, where it's just "index." In French, there's a double meaning from my understanding. Therefore, when you read the text in English, you're missing out on a fair amount of theoretical specificity of what Laplanche is saying.

NE: This is interesting, because I have so many patients who dream about the sea [*mer*], and it's all about the mother [*mère*]. Their associations lead to that. Signifiers are very important, and it is almost certain that the Laplanchian emphasis on signifiers is an *indebtedness* to Lacan. Let us not forget that Laplanche was analyzed by Lacan and was very close to him, before taking a distance from his analytic father. Remember how Laplanche criticizes Lacan's use of the big Other. However, contrary to Freud, he stresses the primacy of the other just like Lacan. There is a clear filiation between Lacan and Laplanche, even though this filiation is denied. I don't really like the official translation of *socius proche* in English. I would translate it to "the small group of intimate others." I think it's more comprehensible in English.

BBT: I went to look it up. This is the precise quote of the English translation: "Of course, it is in 'the social' that the assignment is inscribed, if only in that famous declaration at the beginning of life that is made at the level of the institutional structures of a given society.... It is the little group of closed *socii* of friends and blood relations" (Laplanche, 2011, p. 181)."

NE: "Closed socii of friends and blood relations": Where does that come from? This is a very free translation. In any case, Laplanche underscores the dimension of the social. Among mainstream French psychoanalysts, Laplanche is perhaps the only one who takes into consideration the implication of the social to our subjective construction, and the first European analyst to integrate gender in metapsychology, while the majority of psychoanalysts in Europe argue that gender is an extra-analytic, even an anti-analytic concept. Some very traditional, especially senior French analysts even maintain that the whole field of gender studies is an infantile theory and malady, which claims to be scientific.

Laplanche was innovative probably because he engaged in multiple interdisciplinary dialogues, unlike most of his peers. Let us also recall that Lacan integrated interdisciplinary thinking in his work—philosophy, linguistics, anthropology, and so on. Now I'm thinking that there are stronger Lacanian influences in Laplanche's theory than I had expected. I mentioned before Ferenczi and Margaret Mead, but now I'm thinking about the revision of the Oedipus complex by Lacan. He reversed the direction of the Oedipus complex. Instead of imagining that the child has sexual and hostile drives toward his/her/their parents, Lacan stressed the paramountcy of the mother's desire regarding the child. According to him, the child simply responds to the other's desire. It all comes from the M (O)ther. Having said this, Laplanche is more subtle when he emphasizes the primacy of the other.

BBT: Interesting, but I was wondering if we could go back to countertransference. You mentioned your take on the analyst's transference to work and one's countertransference. However, Laplanche has a very specific stance on countertransference. I'm not sure if one would say that he doesn't care for it, but he doesn't see its utility. Maybe that's pushing it too much. One of the things is that one cannot know their account of countertransference in an analytic session because the session is for the patient and for the patient's material. It's not for the analyst to analyze their own material. I was wondering, how do you think about that theoretically, clinically? Do you use your countertransference clinically? I know you said that you're not just a Laplanchean but also use different theories, depending upon the patient. It's not always just the patient, but the moments that the patient's in and where they're functioning.

NE: Exactly, you're absolutely right. A variety of theories are necessary not only in order to listen to different patients, but also to apprehend different moments of the same treatment. You're absolutely right to nuance this. I have my own perception about countertransference, but at the same time, I have a Laplanchean influence. Laplanche uses *après-coup* in different contexts, but then I take *après-coup* in my own context. Just to remind us of what Laplanche says. He tries to reconstitute the notion of afterwardsness throughout Freud's work. What I really like is the complexification of *après-coup by* Laplanche. He discovers the insufficiency of Strachey's translation of the word….

BBT: "Deferred action."

NE: Yes, I was looking for the German word. Strachey speaks about deferred action and Jung spoke about retrospective action. We have deferred actions and movements from the past to the present, and retroactive movements from the present to the past. Laplanche's major contribution to the concept of *après-coup* is the bidirectional movement of it. We have deferred action and also a retroactive dimension, regredient and progredient movements, regressive and progressive. We have this spiral movement as emphasized by Jonathan House. This spiral movement being a to and fro. The regressive and progressive movement is not obvious in the Freudian corpus.

I'm going to make the connection with countertransference now. The most important thing for me is the intersubjective dimension of *après-coup*. When Freud uses the concept of *après-coup* in the case of the Wolf Man, he focuses on the intrapsychic dimension of post-hoc perspective. That suggests that in an analysis it is possible to reinterpret one's own experiences under the sway of afterwardsness.

That said, is it only about the analysand? No, it is also about the analyst who interprets the analysand's material, thus helping the analysand to give a new meaning to his/her/their experiences. Nevertheless, Freud never takes into consideration the intersubjective dimension of *après-coup*. Contrastingly, Laplanche underscores the intersubjective dimension of *après-coup*. However, he doesn't show specifically how this intersubjective aspect of *après-coup* functions in the transference. In my view, the transference is the ultimate raison d'être of *après-coup* because the analysand is able to give a new meaning to their experiences thanks to the analyst's interventions. The analysand's experiences are constantly reinterpreted, de-translated, and re-translated, thanks to the analyst's interpretations and constructions.

This for me is the fruitfulness of the notion of *après-coup*. We translate our experiences differently every time thanks to the presence of the other. Countertransference is of course, by definition, inscribed in the *après-coup*. We never realize our countertransference in the moment of the session; we always realize or become conscious of countertransference reactions in the *après-coup*. Personally, I can become conscious of my countertransference thanks to the *après-coup* of writing. Because writing for me is like introducing a third, a supervising other. Through writing I realize what I may have missed in the session, what I could have said or not said, what I should have not said. I become conscious of my countertransference thanks to writing, conversations like the one I am having with you right now, exchanges with supervisors or peers, interactions during conferences.

I have to add here that the analyst also gets transformed through and thanks to his/her/their analysands. For instance, I had a very different stance and views from a theoretical point of view about transness. While I always considered myself as a progressive analyst, I was actually reproducing norms and conservative theories despite me. Thanks to the multiple transferences and countertransferences with my trans, queer, and gender-creative patients, I realized that many of the theories which had shaped my listening were outdated and antiquated. Consequently, I had to deconstruct my transference toward traditional psychoanalytic "dogmas", discover new transferences, and cathect new theoretical premises.

That was made through the transference toward my analysands and my countertransference awareness, which was not an automatic process, but that was inscribed in the *après-coup*. It took me many years with different transferential experiences and countertransferential elaborations and working through of my reflections and understandings of my thoughts about gender, transgender, and so on. I came to have a completely different attitude about these topics.

To my knowledge, Laplanche does not apply the intersubjective dimension of *après-coup* in the transference, in the clinical setting. He never gives clinical examples regarding this issue. However, when he comes back to *après-coup* in his paper "Gender, Sex, and the *Sexual*" (2003), Laplanche describes that the child before the adults tries to understand the enigmatic messages transmitted by them. At the same time, the adults before the child reactivate their own infantile sexuality. Accordingly, there is this double movement, this intersubjective scene. I think that this is so precious from a clinical point of view. For instance, in the transference, both the analysand's and the analyst's infantile sexuality are rekindled.

I will give an example. Some years ago, I started working with parents of children or adolescents in transition. What was really fascinating was the emergence of polysexual and polygender dreams and fantasies in the parents, which suggested a revival of their infantile sexuality. In other words, the child's hybridity triggered some overwhelming bisexual, transsexual, and polysexual fantasies. Similarly, the polymorphic infantile sexuality of the analyst who treats a trans patient is likely to be rekindled in the transference.

BBT: How is that not reproduced in the session with the patient or what the patient brings in regarding their gender?

NE: What I can say is there are parts of ourselves that we try to repress, and this is the *Sexual*, the agitation of our repressed infantile sexuality. According to Laplanche, it's not just the social forces that repress the *Sexual*: the ego needs structure and adaptation; hence it tends to regulate the polymorphism of the drives through binary oppositions masculine/feminine, phallic/castrated, etc. The ego needs to put an order to the primitive anarchy of the drives and the chaos of the unconscious. We all have repressed parts of our infantile sexuality; even if we are the most emancipated sexual beings in the world, there are always untranslated remainders of our infantile experiences. I think that in the transference, many patients are more likely to arouse our repressed infantile sexuality. Our countertransference refers to this agitation; it is a manifestation of our overflowing excitement.

Firstly, there is an overexcitement in parents whose children transition. These parents revive many aspects of their infantile stimulations. A mother I had in therapy a few years ago made this connection herself. She said her child's transition made her go back, relive infantile arousals, affects, and emotions, even sexual abuses. She was impressed by the fact that her child's transition triggered an array of sexual dreams (giving blow jobs to men, doing cunnilingus to other women, being endowed with a penis and a vagina, having sexual intercourse with the analyst), and this efflorescence of sexual dreams and fantasies made me realize that the analyst can be aroused in a similar fashion with trans analysands.

Some dreams made her free associate to sexual positions and practices such as 69. She told me, "Oh, your phone number has the number 69." There were massive fantasies which regarded the analyst and that was the aftereffect of her daughter's transition from female-to-male. I realized in the *après-coup* that I was overflown with excitement by this material and that this overwhelming excitation and agitation made me rigid in the sessions and cling on to theory. This was a defense against all this excitation, against the revival of the *Sexual* in the transference.

I think that what Laplanche says about the intersubjective dimension of the *après-coup* is essential: It is not just the child who tries to understand and make meaning of the adults' enigmatic messages, it is not only the child who is overstimulated but also the adult when confronted with the child who reactivates his or her infantile sexuality and re-translates the enigmatic messages he/she/they received during his/her/their childhood. Similarly, it is not only the analysand who is aroused by the analyst's enigma, it is also the analyst who is aroused by the analysand's sexual and gender enigma. Our analysands make us think what we don't want to think about the repressed parts of our sexuality and gender. Remember Judith Butler's notion of gender melancholy, which refers to the amputation of certain erogenous zones in our body due to the taboo of homosexuality. There is indeed a kind of melancholy, and all these melancholically erased parts of ourselves are awakened, aroused, and stirred up through the transference.

This is why we are disturbed; we are troubled. One way to defend ourselves against this rekindlement of repressed excitations is to not listen to the patients. Or, sometimes a sleepiness takes over as a defense mechanism. Or we might clinically mistreat patients by proposing violent, normative, projective, or even delirious interpretations. Because we are not aware that we're agitated, we have the illusion that we propose accurate interpretations, whereas in reality we're struggling with our own agitation and internal violence.

BBT: How does this come up with the clinical vignettes?

NE: What struck me at the beginning of the museum scene vignette was the sentence in parentheses: "I know you don't really like museums and would rather go alone. But I have two tickets for us."

BBT: The boyfriend's statement?

NE: Yes, the boyfriend's statement. I am not sure if I can interpret the latter in the Laplanchean terms of enigmatic message. Here I understand a paradoxical message rather than an enigmatic one. Laplanche evokes in "Gender, Sex, and the *Sexual*" that sometimes we have a contradiction between conscious and unconscious meanings in the messages which emanate from the primordial others. For instance, a father may consciously assign the male gender to his offspring while he expected

> a girl, or even unconsciously wished to penetrate a girl. I believe that Laplanche describes in this example a paradox and not an enigma. Likewise, in the museum scene vignette, we don't have any enigma, but a paradox. Several readings, such as the work by Luiz Carlos Tarelho, have helped me to expand the Laplanchean thinking. Needless to recall that everything in Laplanche is about communication, especially enigmatic communication, which leaves space and freedom for translation, interpretation, and psychic autonomy. Attention however: Laplanche does not only speak about enigmatic signifiers, which are implanted to the child's body ego by the adults, but also intromissive signifiers, that is, messages which are intromitted to the child's psyche, destroy their translational ability, and attack their thought processes. I find it very useful to establish a parallel between these intromissive messages and the double bind theories as described in the seminal paper by Gregory Bateson and his collaborators (1956) "Towards a Theory of Schizophrenia," Harold Searles's (1959) "The Effort to Drive the Other Person Crazy," and the works on paradoxical communication by Didier Anzieu, Paul-Claude Racamier, and René Roussillon.

The child is sometimes confronted with contradictory and self-annihilating messages which are impossible to metabolize and digest. These messages create a paradox, to be distinguished from enigma, which creates space for thinking. Paradox attacks thinking instead, and it might drive somebody crazy. This is why traditionally we associate paradoxical communication with psychosis. Generally, even though paradoxical communication can be found anywhere, it can lead to psychosis indeed if somebody from their primary childhood is confronted constantly and repetitively to paradoxical messages.

To go back to the vignette, I think that what the boyfriend proposed is something paradoxical. To reply or respond to a paradoxical message is difficult. Remember the intromissive messages that do not allow translation. In these cases of intromissive messages, we just reproduce the same message without any translation. The reproduction of the message suggests total submission to the other and the confiscation of one's autonomous thinking. In my view, the analysand in the vignette is irritated. She is unable to say "no" due to the intromissive character of her boyfriend's statement, which may have probably reactivated other intromissive or paradoxical messages that she received when she was a child, hence her difficulty in dealing with the situation. This is probably why she ends up going to the museum with her boyfriend.

I think there is a difficulty in asserting her own voice, in showing her psychic autonomy or, in Laplanche's terms, a difficulty in translating in her own terms what she has received from the other. However, for me, the most important thing is what is not mentioned in the vignette—the fact that the analyst appears to be unconcerned by his/her/their analysand's narrative.

Patients do not speak in analysis as if they were chatting with a friend or another person. They always communicate unconscious messages to the analyst through their narratives. I am referring here to transferential messages. Following this logic, the museum in the first vignette can be seen as a metaphor of psychic life. The exploration of the museum plausibly refers to the exploration of multiple layers of the analysand's past. Accordingly, what she actually says to the analyst is that she is ambivalent about analysis: Does she wish to be accompanied along her associations or does she prefer to explore the museum of her psychic life on her own? Or perhaps she is saying to the analyst that she would prefer him to talk less and let her make interpretations of her own.

Laplanche insists on a very traditional analytic stance of opacity, neutrality, and silence. Remember that this analytic stance was canonical at his time. There are still analysts who barely interpret, speak, or react because they need to accentuate the representation of the analyst as an enigmatic figure. While the analyst's enigma and accentuated neutrality may work well with neurotic patients, this technique is not always efficient; I should rather say that it is even counterproductive with patients with less organized representations or with severely traumatized patients, as Sándor Ferenczi (1933/1949) argued, but also André Green and Howard Levine.

BBT: I want to pull something out and clarify it. I understand the premise of you saying that the analysand might feel ambivalent about the analysis. I understand the piece about the museum and your reference to the traditional analytic stance. My understanding is Laplanche didn't speak very much outside the consulting room nor in the consulting room. I understand the submission to the analyst. However, I became lost on why would the analysand want the analyst to speak less? What communicated that to you?

NE: If we stick to my interpretation that the whole vignette is a transferential message, the fact that she's not fond of museums and when she does attend, she prefers to go alone, she doesn't want to be with her boyfriend/analyst. It's as if she was expressing the need to explore museums on her own, without being parasitized by the other's overwhelming or overpowering presence. She needs to feel that she's analyzing herself and doesn't need the boyfriend/analyst to explore the museum. Or maybe she is telling the analyst that she needs him to be more discrete, more silent, and more enigmatic so that she can do the creative work of translation instead of having him translate for her.

BBT: Understood. What were your thoughts on the second vignette?

NE: For the second vignette, I focused on some signifiers such as engagement and engagement ring. I thought about the ring, but I also thought about box ... box ring. How is this said in English?

BBT: You were correct: "boxing ring."

NE: Yes, exactly, because what happened is like someone punched his nose. This made me think about boxing rings and I thought about the engagement ring. One does not request to reduce the frequency of the analytic sessions without an underlying reason. I read between the lines that this patient had to diminish the frequency of the sessions for defensive reasons. In order to protect himself from the analytic commitment or engagement. He actually disengages himself from the treatment, while at the same time he is ready to be engaged to another person.

For me, these two concomitant things are inextricably linked because we clearly have a case of lateral transference. Laplanche does not extensively develop the phenomenon of lateral transference, but he does mention it in his paper "Transference: Its Provocation by the Analyst" in *The Unfinished Copernican Revolution*. Lateral transference refers to a displacement of the transference to outside the analytic space. For instance, the analysand may fall in love with a person right after or shortly after the analysis begins.

A lateral transference is a kind of protection from the analytic commitment or from what happens in analysis. According to some authors, lateral transference is an acting out, an action beyond the analytic space. Something revives a primary trauma which is not represented, or which is very weakly represented. Because this archaic trauma is not represented, the analysand unconsciously does something outside the analysis.

For me, the analysand in the second vignette is intensely defending himself against something. It seems vital for him at this stage of the treatment to diminish the frequency of the sessions. On a conscious level, he believes that it is a matter of money. This is actually a leitmotif in the analysis of almost all patients. However, the financial argument is a resistance to analysis. Lateral transference is also a resistance.

Let me quote Laplanche: "Lateral transference, acting out, an infidelity to the analytic relation—what are we to do with this? It may be drawn back into that relation, interpreted, in sum, as *a transference of the transference:* 'What you could not, did not wish to, tell me, you have signified, enacted, somewhere else'" (Laplanche & Thurston, 518). Laplanche says here that the analytic stance when we have a lateral transference is not to confront the patient directly as the analyst in the vignette. Instead of interpreting this, I would have rather left it open because I think that this is a fragile patient. Or perhaps I would use an interpretation in the form of a question so as to avoid the potentially traumatizing verticality of classical interpretation.

In confronting him directly, it functions as an intromissive message that perforates the psychophysiological skin of the patient. Remember Laplanche: While the implantation of enigmatic messages has both traumatic and structuring effects, intromission, which is the violent variant of implantation, dismantles the translational capacity. That's to say, anything that has to do with representation and symbolization. Intromission suggests the perforation of the skin ego (or body ego) of the child/analysand. In this case, the analyst's confrontation functions literally as an "Intromitted" message. Bion (2013), who has a rich clinical experience with psychosis, describes a patient who received the analyst's interpretation as a bullet that intruded their body. In the vignette, we have something complex due to the lateral transference. The latter occurs when there is too much aggressiveness towards the analyst.

I find useful the openings of the Laplanchean framework by Christophe Dejours, who argues that when we have intromissive messages during childhood, in the *après-coup* of adolescence, we have different forms of actions instead of mental processes: delinquency, criminal acts (acting out), or psychosomatic breakdowns (acting in). Since the person is unable to assimilate or metabolize something intrusive, they engage in actions. One of these actions which suggest the failure of psychic work can be the psychosomatic symptom. The nosebleed for me is like a punch of the nose. Language, symbols, or metaphors collapse into literal action. It is as if the analyst threw a punch at the patient's nose. What is also interesting is that the analysand bleeds everywhere, including the analytic couch. He makes the couch dirty. In my view, this is a hint to the analysand's aggressivity toward the analyst. It's important to clarify that this symptom is not a hysterical symptom expressed through the body, which involves representation and symbolization. In the vignette, it is clearly something which was poorly represented or not symbolized at all. This is why there is a discharge in the soma.

BBT: I noticed that you pay very close attention to metaphors and metonymies, or one could say condensation and displacement. What theoretical place are you drawing from to listen in that way?

NE: Your observation is about my being sensitive to signifiers, to metaphors and metonymies, which I think comes from Freud, Lacan, and Laplanche. Because firstly, I'm influenced by *The Interpretation of Dreams*.

BBT: I was also going to say you have a literature background, don't you?

NE: Yes. I have done classics and then a doctorate in modern Greek literature. I became a clinical psychologist and psychoanalyst some years afterward. I think that it is interesting that you bring my background here because I was always fond of stories, tales, signifiers, metaphors, and metonymies. I pay attention to signifiers because of my literary background and also because of my own analysis. I am always fascinated by dreams and their usage of language. Playing with words and homonyms. For instance, I had an analysand who dreamt of a pair of blue jeans. The blue jeans were so persistent in his narrative. That, of course, was a symbol of his youth and his nonchalance. I had this epiphany and thought about the melancholy that the patient had about his hereditary illness. Therefore, I thought about "blue jeans" as "blue genes", that is melancholic genes, and when I proposed this to the patient, he started crying because my interpretation uncovered his denied feelings about his genetic condition. That was an influence from *The Interpretation of Dreams*. Of course, the question of signifiers is something that we owe to Lacan and Laplanche's theory of enigmatic signifiers. Laplanche is influenced by Lacan, of course, but what is interesting about Laplanche is that he expands the sense of signifier beyond language. With Lacan we only have linguistic signifiers, while with Laplanche we have pre-linguistic and para-linguistic signifiers. Any kind of message, anything semiotic, any kind of infra/preverbal message. This is extremely interesting!

I think that this second vignette of yours is exciting. One can meditate and think about every single detail regarding the engagement, the engagement ring, and spending money for other things than the analysis. I wanted to say that, for me, the intromissive piece and the psychosomatic symptom response to the analyst's interpretation are related to this lateral transference. This lateral transference often conceals unmetabolized and represented states or traumas and deals with aggressiveness and hostility. We can make correlations between this aggressivity and some other elements of the vignette such as the fact that he bled all over the analytic couch.

I think that the patient in your third vignette has experienced the analyst's interpretation as a serious separation. Maybe a kind of tearing up his skin, in a way. Perhaps I'm extrapolating too much. However, there is this rage of feeling separated, and there are feelings of isolation. For the analysand, it was as though you were pushing them away and creating further feelings of isolation with the pain they were already feeling.

BBT: The reaction was quite disproportionate to what was happening. Clearly, there's a strong indication that it's a transferential reaction.

NE: Sure.

BBT: I understood it as a moment where one can think about hollowed-out transference.

NE: Okay.

BBT: Hollowed-out transference versus filled-in transference. I could have said something to the effect of, "You're concerned about me going off and separating from you the way your mother and father did." The person's mother and father were frequently traveling, and they were left with the nanny. I could say something like that. I didn't. I don't generally say things like that. But instead, we discussed the comment itself while the person was in a frenzy of rage with me. Often, when I ask people who think with Laplanche's ideas about the hollowed-out transference, they give me the textbook response. It both is and isn't that.

NE: As I said regarding the first vignette, Laplanche had a quite traditional concept of the analytic stance, which for me is too traditional, and caught in the French tradition of analytic mutism. Analytic silence, as Laplanche conceptualized it, is against even the Freudian argument about proposing to the patient a construction after a certain time. Not just an interpretation, but a construction, that is, a synthetic view of the patient's past. Laplanche is firmly against any synthesis, any binding that comes from the analyst.

For Laplanche, analysis is all about decomposition and deconstruction. He argues that all should come from the analysand. The analysand should deconstruct, construct, and reconstruct. However, the analyst should never propose constructions. Again, for Laplanche, he's referencing the etymological sense of analysis as dissolution, decomposition, and deconstruction.

I think Laplanche was much more subtle and refined than Lacan's argument that the analyst should play dead. However, when he emphasizes that the analyst should never be helping the analysand to construct, but only to deconstruct, he implicitly argues that the analysts should be very succinct in their interventions.

The Laplanchean *style* in the session is to be economical and to count your words. Not to say too much, mainly draw the analysand's attention to specific signifiers. My clinical experience makes me think that there is perhaps an overemphasis by Laplanche on the primacy of the other. I am also aware of something which was referred to me by a colleague of mine at the *Université Paris Cité* Department of Psychoanalytic Studies, which was founded by Laplanche. This colleague visited Laplanche's château and worked with him closely and claims that shortly before his death, Laplanche thought that he may have placed too much emphasis on the primacy of the other in his theoretical constructions about the emergence of subjectivity. I am not sure if it is a fantasy by the person who told me this, or if it is something that Laplanche really said.

Either way, it might be challenging for us to think that everything emanates from the other. It leaves out that children come into the world with any drive. Even though I believe that the role of the object is of paramount importance, I think that there are some elements which are innate. Laplanche seems to imply that the child is like a tabula rasa, a blank screen, and it's the other's enigma which gives rise to the drive to translate. The very notion of drive is consubstantial to the other's presence.

For me, this conception, although I find it interesting, in that it gives space to otherness and to what happens in primary interactions and the role of the objects, it's as if we regress to a pre-Freudian conception of the child as a totally innocent creature. Unlike Jean-Jacques Rousseau, who believed that the child was born entirely pure and innocent, Freud illustrated the child's inherent polymorphous perversity. Laplanche seems to efface this endogenous drivenness when he argues that the infant does not have any unconscious and that the emergence of the drives is the outcome of the others' enigmatic messages. I think that it is an error to overlook the implication of constitutional factors.

In my view, there are some proto-psychic elements from the very beginning, a kind of primary drivenness. Otherwise, I have difficulty in understanding how the child translates the adults' messages if he or she doesn't carry anything to start out with. Before any translation, before any adult message, there must be something already there.

I think that the infant tries to communicate something to the adult as soon as they come to life. It's not just the adult's response that makes drives emerge. I think that there is something more dialectical between the child's drives and the object's responsiveness (or unresponsiveness).

Having said this, I consider Laplanche to be a nonbinary thinker par excellence. He was indeed very much attracted by the theories of multiplicities and plurality. In his own theory, Laplanche introduces a third element, that of thirdness; and this is the element of the message, the message that circulates within the adult/child dyad.

Laplanche was probably trying to escape from Freud's binary thinking. Going further, Laplanche defines psychic reality as a third order of reality parallel to psychological and material reality. For me, this is another conceptual triangulation and, also, the concept of the *Sexual*, which comes from his paper "Gender, Sex, and the *Sexual*."

Laplanche in this paper goes beyond the conundrum of sex/gender and complexifies the discussion by articulating a third term, the *Sexual*, which is his "translation" of Freud's polymorphous perversity. Interestingly, Laplanche understands the masculine/feminine, phallic/castrated polarities as a translation of the original overwhelming plurality of gender messages. More specifically, Laplanche considers binaries to be a bulwark against the initial over-exciting and over-exceeding polymorphism of the drives, with masculine/feminine and phallic/castrated polarities bringing order to the erratic anarchy of the unconscious. I can recall Frances Tustin (1990), who highlights certain primary oppositions (hard/soft, hot/cold, dry/wet), which serve the infant as "landmarks" in the original chaos of instinctual impulses. The common thread of these theories is the structuring virtues of binaries, their potential of regulation of the chaotic too-muchness of the drives. Perhaps this is why we have the perpetuation of gender binary throughout so many generations.

Although gender emerges before the recognition of anatomical sex difference, it does not constitute a primary formation, since it is preceded by the primitive anarchy of the drives. Which drives? Laplanche calls this unbound drivenness *le sexual*, which refers to pregenital and paragenital drives. Despite the divergence of different theories, gender seems to bind and regulate this overwhelming drivenness of the unconscious. Accordingly, the child's assimilation of messages such as "You're a little boy" or "You're a little girl" can function as an infantile theory capable of giving order to the original chaos of the drives and bringing unity and continuity to the fragmented identity of the child. This is why gender, which supports self-image and apparently prevents body shapes from vanishing in the mirror – I mean the mirroring other, and by vanishing, I mean disappearing in the other's gaze – is a matter of life and death for some analysands. Hence comes the risk of going astray in violent, projective, or even delusional interpretations if we fail to sufficiently work through the death-associated elements that circulate in the transference behind the mask of the masculine and the feminine.

Overall, I would like to stress that Laplanchean epistemology is a nonbinary epistemology; it rather constitutes a post-binary epistemology. Another thing that I really like is that the translational model by Laplanche is synonymous with becoming.

BBT: Are you using becomingness in the Deleuzian sense?

NE: Yes. For me, the concept of translation is very dynamic. It is a conception of the human being seen and considered as in everlasting transition. Laplanche's translational model actually refers to a constant reshaping of human subjectivity. There's an ongoing process of translation, de-translation, and re-translation, which creates something very fluid and transformative in terms of identity.

We have vertical messages that come from the adults, from the adults/child asymmetrical communication. In fact, Laplanche highlights in his own way the verticality of identifications, which was put forward by classical psychoanalysis. However, if we read Laplanche's various texts carefully, we see that he takes into consideration horizontal messages as well. These are messages that emanate from culture and society (Laplanche, 1992, p. 416).[2] I think this is essential, especially nowadays, when horizontality is more important since it competes with verticality.

Adolescents are confronted with many horizontal messages. Those from groups of peers, the internet, social media, Instagram, Facebook, Twitter, and so on. The discourse of the other is not just the discourse of the adults, the messages by the *socius proche*. It is also the extended *socius*. There are many horizontal messages that come from the internet and social media. Accordingly, Laplanche introduces the concept of the mytho-symbolic. A concept I like very much.

The mytho-symbolic assists translation. I think this makes Laplanche contemporary. The child, and later, the adolescent, translates the enigmatic signifiers using social and cultural codes, "pre-formed narratives," to quote Laplanche, which are available in their time. The mytho-symbolic is not something static, fixed, universal, but something contingent, dynamic, which transforms itself. Translation and re-translation are an ongoing process. We might understand the evolution of someone's sexuality or gender in these terms. We can understand gender transitions, de-transitions, or re-transitions as a consequence of this process of de-translation and re-translation that also take into consideration social and cultural narratives.

Subjectivity is not just about early identifications, as in many orthodox metapsychologies, where it is simply the child who identifies to the parent. There are many vertical and horizontal messages and identifications in the Laplanchean model. This is why I find the Laplanchean model enriching and I consider transness as the paradigm of translation and psychoanalytic becomingness.

This is something that I see in my clinical practice, and this is how I would articulate this becomingness with the Laplanchean notion of *après-coup*. Not just what I think about myself, but what I think about myself in relation to the other, in relation to what the other tells me, or what the other signifies to me, or suggests to me. This other is not just the parent, it's also my group of peers, it's also society; it is the analyst as well, whose interpretations and constructions can make me change and get transformed.

I also like that Laplanche takes into consideration the idiosyncratic dimension of translation. We have multiple translations, re-translations, and so on. Laplanche takes into consideration the fact that two subjects might receive the same messages. However, the way they are going to metabolize, interpret them, depends on their idiosyncratic disposition and temperament. There is always an irreducibly singular translation, inscription, metabolization, and assimilation.

The translational model of becomingness and the fact that Laplanche is a nonbinary thinker and invokes conceptual triangulation brings me to interdisciplinarity. I would like to make the connection with a question about the Laplanchean *style* of research in psychoanalysis. I like Laplanche's unfinished Copernican revolution and desire to free psychoanalysis from ipsocentrism and solipsistic closure. There is an epistemological dialogism and polyphony in Laplanche.

Mainstream French psychoanalysis is not only fixated on a solipsistic psychic reality but also on a narcissistic monodisciplinary thinking. I am not certain about the United States, but definitely here in France, psychoanalysis resists the knowledge coming from other disciplines. That said, Laplanchean-*style* research in psychoanalysis is inherently interdisciplinary. Laplanche constantly engaged in disciplinary otherness. Other disciplines such as philosophy—his original theoretical background—anthropology, literature, feminist studies, and gender theory, etc. I also appreciate the fact that he engages in dialogue with non-French psychoanalysts, hence with metapsychological concepts coming from different linguistic traditions.

I consider his work as a vigorous dialogue with Freud, Lacan, Ferenczi, Klein, Winnicott, Green, etc. Laplanchean-*style* research is inherently polyphonic. Polyphonic in the sense of Mikhail Bakhtin, the Russian literary critic and philosopher who spoke about multivoiced dialogue and the transformative power of dialogism. When we speak nowadays about interdisciplinary knowledge and thinking, there is the danger of conceptual approximation. However, in Laplanche's case, it's completely different. While he encourages dialogue with other disciplines, Laplanche is extremely rigorous and emphasizes the specificities of psychoanalysis as an independent epistemological field.

BBT: Apparently, his study groups were such that they would discuss anthropology and all sorts of other disciplines. He was very well versed in them.

NE: How do I conceive a Laplanchean *style* of research in psychoanalysis? I am, of course, influenced by my own background, and by the fact that I am in the department that was founded by Laplanche. It is important to note that he founded this department because he needed to create a different space from psychoanalytic institutes in order to promote psychoanalytic research in academia. He believed that there were too many splittings, discords, and uncreative disputes within psychoanalytic institutes. He envisaged the university as a *third* space. One where we could have proper, independent thinking about research in psychoanalysis. This is how he conceived of and introduced not just psychoanalysis at the university, but he later created a doctorate in psychoanalysis, which continues into today.

Laplanche advocated for an extraterritoriality principle, both in clinical practice and in the field of research. It is a particularity of the French IPA model, the extraterritoriality principle. This is the signature of the *Association psychanalytique de France* (APF) in France. Actually, the founders of the APF, and among them Laplanche, insisted on the necessity of abolishing the training analysis.

APF differentiated itself from other IPA institutes by insisting on the exclusion of any institutional interference into the candidate's analysis. According to this model, analysis should be an independent, completely free space. The analyst of the candidate should not interfere with the person's training. In concrete terms, extraterritoriality means that the analyst of a person wishing to undertake training would never again be asked in any way whatsoever by their peers to give an opinion on the person's background and aptitudes. Nor would the analyst have to accompany the person through the process.

Personal analysis remains the primary condition for commitment to training, and no one other than the candidate himself will be held accountable for it. The APF welcomes candidates for training without regard to their original couch, which is to say without their analyst's status or membership in any particular society being a prerequisite of selection. This is the extraterritoriality principle of clinical practice. For Laplanche, the university is an antidote to the rigidity and univocal thinking of psychoanalytic institutes. Perhaps there is a kind of idealization of the university by Laplanche.

BBT: You have mentioned separately that the Platonic dialogues are part of Laplanche's epistemology. I know he studied with Jean Hyppolite, who was a Hegelian scholar. Laplanche's writing, his essays, are generally very dialectical. They start with a thesis, move to the antithesis, then to a sort of synthesis, which is where he introduces his thought. Can you say more about this conceptual triangulation?

NE: The crux of my point is the following: in order to integrate otherness, we must integrate a third-party function; we have to be able to triangulate. I will go into greater depth on this. Start from what is clinically relevant, because we do have patients who cannot triangulate or have a difficulty in triangulating. Initially, there is the dyad relationship between the infant and the primordial other. Traditionally, we have the initial dyad of an infant and, let me say mother just in order to be simpler to elaborate. The child needs to be able to create autonomous thinking in order to be able to symbolize and separate themselves from this initial object. In Lacanian thinking, it is the father who functions as a third party, necessary to separate the infant from its mother. However, it is because at the time, the caregiving process was synonymous to the mother, and the third entity separate to it was synonymous to the father.

However, nowadays we have men who have a caregiving function and women who have the third-party function, the one that separates the infant from this initial dyad. Lacan said that it was not the physical presence of the father that created this separation, but the presence of the father in the mother's mind. There are things that can occur to derail this process. This will cause the infant to remain entrapped in this duality, and they will have difficulty in triangulating, in integrating another person, thirdness.

I like to say thirdness, internalization of thirdness, triangulation, the capacity to triangulate or to integrate something other than my mother's desire for me. In order to be able to have this autonomy and free thinking, one must integrate the fact that one's mother, or the person that deals with me at the very beginning, desires something beyond me. This is how I integrate the third-party function, otherwise I remain entrapped in this solipsistic and undifferentiated dyad.

Laplanche speaks of signifiers and translations. He is opposed to psychosexual developmental stages. He instead conceives of a dynamic model of enigmatic signifiers to be translated and this constant and endless translational process goes beyond any kind of developmental ideal and axiological norm. However, what I was saying about conceptual triangulation is that if we remain confined into our narcissistic disciplinary enclosure, it is as if we are not capable of integrating otherness.

Conceptual triangulation for me is about being able to have a transference toward other fields of theory, disciplines, which releases us from the solipsistic psychoanalytic thinking and enclosures. Laplanche discusses this at length in the essay, which is also the name of the book that contains the paper, *Unfinished Copernican Revolution*.

BBT: Could you say a little about the category of the message and psychic reality?

NE: It is important to stress the third category of reality, the reality of the message. He is constantly in search of a third space or a third term or a third order. The reality of the message is that psychic space between material and psychological reality.

BBT: Even Laplanche's *après-coup* is a third because he's temporally going in two directions—a movement from the present to the past, which then propels the past into the future in a simultaneous spiral. He's not choosing the first direction or the second direction.

NE: I've never thought of *après-coup* in these terms, but I think you're absolutely right. Because instead of deciding between deferred action and retroaction, as we said before, he complexifies this movement, and it's not just deferred action or retroaction. The image of the spiral is a highly complex movement. For me, thirdness in the sense of Laplanche is synonymous to complexity and rigor. A Laplanchean *style* is one of rigor.

Notes

1 See Burkhalter (2018).
2 See this quote: "If we accept the relationship to the enigma of the other as the fundamental dimension of the transference, then perhaps before the analysis or after the analysis, the major place of transference, *the 'ordinary' transference, should be located in the multipolar relationship to culture*, to creation or, more precisely, to the *cultural message*."

Bibliography

Anzieu, D. (1986). Paradoxical transference. *Contemporary Psychoanalysis, 22*(4), 520–547. https://doi.org/10.1080/00107530.1986.10746144

Bakhtin, M. (1984). *Problems of Dostoevsky's poetics* (C. Emerson, Trans.). University of Minnesota Press.

Bateson, G., Jackson, D. D., Haley, J., & Weakland, J. (1956). Toward a theory of schizophrenia. *Behavioral Science, 1*(4), 251–264. https://doi.org/10.1002/bs.3830010402

Bion, W. R. (2013). Attacks on linking. *The Psychoanalytic Quarterly, 82*(2), 285–300. https://doi.org/10.1002/j.2167-4086.2013.00029.x

Burkhalter, T. (2018). Masculinity as a gendered form of desire: Laplanche and enigmatic seduction. *Studies in Gender and Sexuality, 19*(3), 217–230.

Butler, J. (1990). *Gender trouble: Feminism and the subversion of identity*. Routledge.

Calich, J. C. (2006). Pour "faire travailler" la topique laplanchienne. *Psychiatrie française, 37*(3), 34–44.

Dejours, C. (1986). *Le corps entre biologie et psychanalyse*. Payot.

Deleuze, G., & Guattari, F. (1983). *Anti-oedipus: Capitalism and schizophrenia*. University of Minnesota Press.
Deleuze, G., & Guattari, F. (1987). *A thousand plateaus: Capitalism and schizophrenia*. University of Minnesota Press.
Ferenczi, S. (1933/1949). Confusion of tongues between adults and the child. *International Journal of Psychoanalysis*, 30, 225–230.
Freud, S. (1900). *The interpretation of dreams*. SE 4.
Gernet, I. (2020). Théorie de la séduction généralisée et théorie du sens: À propos des obstacles au travail de penser. In H. Tessier (Ed.), *Psychanalyse et théorie du sens: Un dialogue entre la pensée de Jean Laplanche et la sémiotique* (pp. 189–218). PUF. https://doi.org/10.3917/puf.tessi.2021.01.0189
Green, A. (1999). *The work of the negative*. Free Association Books.
Laplanche, J. (1992). Du transfert: Sa provocation par l'analyste [Transference: Its provocation by the analyst]. In *La révolution copernicienne 1967–1992* [Essays in Otherness] (pp. 417–438). PUF.
Laplanche, J. (2005). *Essays on otherness*. Routledge.
Laplanche, J. (2007). *Sexual: La sexualité élargie au sens freudien*. PUF.
Laplanche, J. (2008). *La révolution copernicienne inachevée. 1967–1992*. PUF.
Laplanche, J. (2011). *Freud and the sexual*. The Unconscious in Translation.
Laplanche, J., & House, J. (2016). *New foundations for psychoanalysis*. The Unconscious in Translation.
Laplanche, J., & Mehlman, J. (2015). *Between seduction and inspiration: Man*. The Unconscious in Translation.
Laplanche, J., & Thurston, L. (2020). *The unfinished Copernican revolution: Selected works, 1967–1992*. The Unconscious in Translation.
Levine, H. B. (2021). *Affect, representation and language*. Routledge.
Racamier, P.-C. (2014). On narcissistic perversion. *The International Journal of Psychoanalysis, 95*(1), 119–132. https://doi.org/10.1111/1745-8315.12111
Rousseau, J.-J., & Scott, J. T. (2014). *The major political writings of Jean-Jacques Rousseau: The two discourses and social contract*. The University of Chicago Press.
Roussillon, R. (2013). The function of the object in the binding and unbinding of the drives. *International Journal of Psychoanalysis, 94*(2), 257–276. https://doi.org/10.1111/j.1745-8315.2012.00651.x
Searles, H. F. (1959). The effort to drive the other person crazy—An element in the aetiology and psychotherapy of schizophrenia. *British Journal of Medical Psychology, 32*(1), 1–18. https://doi.org/10.1111/j.2044-8341.1959.tb00463.x
Tarelho, L. C. (1998). *Paranoïa et théorie de la séduction généralisée*. PUF.
Tustin, F. (1990). *The protective shell in children and adults*. Routledge.

9 Avgi Saketopoulou

NYU Postdoctoral Program in Psychotherapy and Psychoanalysis, New York City, USA

Bryan Batista-Thomas: Did any of the questions stand out to you?

Avgi Saketopoulou: I really love your asking after a Laplanchean *style* as opposed to speaking to a Laplanchean *method* or a Laplanchean *technique*. In my opinion, the term "*style*" captures more accurately a sensibility distinctive to a Laplanchean way of listening and of being in the room. That sensibility permeates some of your questions, like when you ask: What are the ethics of a Laplanchean *style*? And how does this relate to metapsychology, clinical practice, and culture?

For me, a Laplanchean *style* is inseparable from thinking about psychoanalytic ethics, which means that a Laplanchean *style* is not a set way of being—otherwise, the theory would become too sclerotic, too constrained, and not pliable to new translations.[1] That would contradict what I see as the most basic principle of Laplanchean thinking—that everything remain open, re-workable, subject to new interpretations, which is to say, that it is always possible in the après-coup for new possibilities of subjectivation to emerge. It is this that makes a Laplanchean *style* inseparable from ethics, that the Laplanchean ethos insists on the ongoing possibility of transmutations of ideas, as long as the basic principles are respected. And that requires that one establish—and tolerate, the latter being a more demanding task—a non-dominating relationship with the otherness in oneself, the otherness in the other, even in the otherness of the theory itself.

To some degree or another, all psychoanalytic schools engage the question of ethics. But here I am not thinking of ethics as concerning rules that might prevent a treatment from going awry, or ethics as pertaining to the moral code of what should not occur (e.g., an ethical transgression)—a distinction between deontology and ethics, which Scarfone (2023) has illuminated. In Laplanchean thinking, ethics, and thus *style*, concern *how* one sits with a patient and that calls up one's relationship to one's own and the other's

DOI: 10.4324/9781032670287-10

enigma. From this angle, a Laplanchean *style* is also inevitably attentive to issues of agency and autonomy—though by "agency" and "autonomy," I am not referring to the neoliberal understandings of a subject that "freely" selects from a range of consumerist options. I mean it, rather, in the way that Laplanche describes the question of response and responsibility (Laplanche & Mehlman, 2015). This is an autonomy that encompasses our response to the ineliminable otherness of the other and to the irreducible otherness in ourselves, to our own sexual unconscious. Autonomy in this sense is not about breaking free of constraints but about how the subject mythologizes herself precisely via such constraints, *by means* of these constraints, how one answers to the constraint (e.g., the constraint that the mytho-symbolic also imposes) and not how one answers for oneself or on behalf of oneself (as, for example, when we say that someone is advocating for themselves).

In *Gender Without Identity,* a book I co-authored with Dr. Ann Pellegrini and which leans heavily on Laplanchean theory, we describe this strange kind of agency as the queer agency of the unconscious to capture the odd quality of something that proceeds *from* the self (and is, therefore, "ours") but is not *of* the self (and is, therefore, always in a decentered relationship to our ego, to our sense of ourselves).

BBT: You are speaking in terms of a Laplanchean *style* being more attentive to agency and autonomy, and you made a link between answering *to* and answering *for*, thereby starting to address the question of a Laplanchean ethics. I'm wondering, what exactly do you mean by agency and autonomy? How does that relate to clinical work?

AS: In everyday conversations, we usually think of agency as something that's proceeding from a centered self where you, as the sovereign agent, may select this or refuse that. But if we think of agency as issuing from an interior center (a true self, a self-possessed nucleus, and so on), we will miss that all agency is allocentric, that is, that agency proceeds from conditions we did not choose and could not—perhaps *would* not—have chosen, and makes use of materials (from the mytho-symbolic, in crafting identifications and counteridentifications, etc.) that were not of our making, many of which we might have never even selected had we been given the chance. For me, what Laplanche helps us see is that the subject's autonomy is not about independence from others or separateness from our circumstance; it inheres in the subject's capacity to translate, to treat the enigma of the other's otherness to us as well as to themselves to produce something new. It gives us a way, that is, to see that agency is not about some imaginary independence from the world and from others but is crafted precisely in response to our interdependence on one another, even in ways that we might not have wanted, and to our existence in a wider historical and political world we did not choose and cannot control.

On this point, I should say, that from early on my study of Laplanche has always been very deeply entwined with my study of Piera Aulagnier (1984). Aulagnier fleshes out a point which is, I think, implicitly present in Laplanche bringing it more into the light: The fact that one always translates by making use of mytho-symbolic materials means that translational codes are by nature restrict*ed*, and thus, also, restrict*ive*. This is because the myths and symbols that are critical to the translational process and which are always already derived from the sociopolitical world[2] are absolutely necessary for the infant to convert the formlessness of the enigmatic into something that has a form, to treat it and, thus, "coat" it with meaning. Every enabling possibility for translation, that is, for symbolization and meaning-making, is an opening into something albeit restrictedly so, within bounds and limits. There's no way around that fact and we encounter a related idea in Laplanche when he insists that every translational movement simultaneously occasions repression. However, to stay with Aulagnier's formulation, all such codes are necessarily restrictive in that they are not infinite and in that their offering therefore also participates in a kind of violence that she called *the violence of interpretation*. These codes, as I expand on in *Sexuality Beyond Consent*, are not neutral; they are themselves suffused with violence, encompassing in them entire lifeworlds that the infant cannot modify, because already swirled in the codes themselves are the prejudices and power relations that subtend them. Not just gender codes per se, but, also, the sexism, patriarchy, and transphobia that subtend them; not just race, but racism, anti-Blackness, and white supremacy, and so on.

As I said, I can't think of Laplanche without Aulagnier, which makes my Laplanche a bit idiomatic—and that's also because I read him through and with trans studies and queer of color critique. But, let's not go there right now. What I am trying to say, to return to agency, is that translation is an exercise of autonomy that necessarily proceeds from within a scene of constraint. Laplanche's theory helps us pay attention to this kind of non-personal, non-subjective restrictiveness; not to the restrictions we are subjected to by individuals (a parent, a lover, a teacher, a boss) or even by the State, but to the restrictions that are inadvertently built into the translating process. For something to become psychically represented, it has to lean on and fabulate from these codes—codes that are both limit*ed* and limit*ing*.

From that angle, the mytho-symbolic is both indispensable to translational activity, but it also implicitly limits *how* something can become psychically intelligible, which shape and form it will take to acquire the property of representation and of legibility. Autonomy, for me, then, is about translation: It has to do with how the raw materials used for translation (materials that exist in the mytho-symbolic and, hence, we have to add, draw also from the sociopolitical realm) are assembled idiomatically—though, again, language fails here because the word "assembled" could be read to imply a centered self, when this process proceeds from a perch that, in Laplanche's formulation, the ego does not command (2015). As a response to being breached by the other, by the other's otherness, translation is always an allocentric process:

Its productions, as I said earlier, do not originate *from* the self, but they are nevertheless *of* the self. It's the latter that gives translation its strange quality of what we can clumsily, with all the above caveats, call agency or autonomy.

BBT: You used the word "subject" a couple times, but then you also said not a centered self. You're simultaneously talking about something that feels displaced or diffuse and at the same time referring to a subject. What are you referring to in Laplanche's theory?

AS: The particular term Laplanche uses for this is "the apparatus of the soul." It's not a term he uses in a quotidian sense, but what he describes as the soul is what I was essentially referring to by the term "subject". For him, the word "soul" does not have its usual religious connotations; he uses it in a more encompassing way to speak about going beyond the way we usually use the term *subject*, the latter leaving out complex operations that have to do with the sexual unconscious, that go beyond one's subjectivity per se, or one's positionality (e.g., race or gender), and that extend beyond inscribed experiences and ego processes. It also goes beyond the secondarily repressed unconscious with its inaccessible but nevertheless represented contents. For him, the apparatus of the soul refers to all these elements *plus* the unrepresented unconscious, which, for him, is sexual through and through. I am using the term "subject" to refer to what he would think of as the soul; the term soul does not appeal to me for various reasons, but I thank you for giving me an opportunity to clarify what I meant.

BBT: I wanted to go back to the mytho-symbolic. You brought up in some ways how the mytho-symbolic functions as a set of limits with their conditions for the soul of the subject to be able to make translations. One of the things that, if I remember correctly, you said that—I'm going to use "individual"—an individual has a mytho-symbolic system that's more encompassing, has more agency, and more autonomy. Can you speak a little bit more about that? Are we talking simply about education? Are we talking about time, changes in culture?

AS: It would be inaccurate, in my opinion, to conclude that if one grows up in a more liberal society, that will necessarily make translations freer, less constrained. That is because, from a metapsychological perspective, autonomy has less to do with the availability of more translational possibilities (aka, a wider mytho-symbolic domain and being exposed to/better educated about it) and more to do with the capacity to exercise translational variety and not be punished for it, e.g., with one's primary objects not exercising undue control over how a child translates (what Laplanche called "intromission"), or when some translations are sanctioned by the social environment (e.g., the suppression of trans experiences over cis ones). It's important to be able to translate without pressure or consequence (the latter being a different form of pressure), that primary objects do not have a controlling impact in how the infant translates. As I was saying, to translate, one must draw from existing translational codes in the mytho-symbolic realm and this has to do with how what's available in the cultural surround is conducted to the child *by the adult*; this conduction always carries the adult's own imprint, inflecting the code with the adult's psychic complexion, including, and especially, that of their sexual unconscious. In other words, even in the same culture, codes don't reach all of us in the same way, nor do we use or translate them necessarily the same way—and this is part of what gives each of us our singularity. But my point is that cultures with wider ranges of mytho-symbolic codes do not produce subjects with more agency, even though they *may* enable the becoming of more variable subjects—and that's an important distinction to make.

BBT: It sounds like you're talking about inspiration.

AS: How so?

BBT: I'm thinking in relation to one's response and interaction with enigma and what one does with it. To be set free almost in a way to do something creative with their translations.

AS: "Creativity" is a word that I am hesitant about but if you are saying that translation can be creative in the sense of not just reproducing something, but generating something new, then I would absolutely agree with you. The reason I would not use the word "creativity" is that what is deemed creative is usually also what is either socially utile or socially acceptable when translation can also generate other things—things that may be seen as deviations or malformations—as is the case, for example, with atypical genders or with sexual desires that are unpalatable even among more open-minded communities. So, there is no guarantee that what arises out of translation will be seen as creative, even as it is "created" by the subject (I am using "subject" here as discussed above). Whatever may be churned out of these translational processes comes to feel one's own precisely *because* it arises out of this very personal operation (the queer agency of the unconscious), but that does not mean that it will always be regarded as a creative outcome—sometimes it may even be unwanted by one's environment or even be seen as destructive!

BBT: This makes me think of clinical practice and what we are doing in the consulting room. It is not educating a patient nor reparenting. What's happening then, do you think?

AS: I agree that we are not reparenting nor are we educating. I'm going to talk about the way I understand psychoanalysis and how I try to practice it via my study of Laplanche. I say try, because I think that doing psychoanalytic work is a constant effort to wrest something from oneself (the clinician's apparatus of the 'soul'). For me, psychoanalysis is neither about mastering a technique nor is it about the analyst absenting herself as some, more classical models might espouse. I think that part of what we're doing most of the time through our interventions is to try to create the conditions for some of the patient's clasped bindings to become less firm, causing them to "blink" so to speak (to use a term from Scarfone, 2023). Bindings that begin to blink may come undone, bringing about the ego's rhexis. I've argued in my work that such a process is anguishing, but that is the path for psychic transformation. Especially so in egoic domains that have become too stiff and inelastic, what Laplanche calls "death by the ego," where things are overly settled this kind of work, the work of analysis, of deconstructing rather than of synthesizing, can be life-changing. We've all sat with patients who have a persuasive story of their origins, stories about who they are, stories of which they are convinced and which may even convince the analyst. I am thinking, for example, of a pedophilic patient I worked with in a maximum security setting, who had a very compelling theory of his sexual attractions to children which had to do with an identification with his abusive parents—this is an example of what I mean about how our patients' self-theorizing may be convincing to us, too. In a psychoanalytic treatment, however, it is less a question of whether these translations/self-theorizations are accurate or not but also what work they do and what they settle, what they resist: How much they tie down, what they stall, what happens in an encounter that disrupts the psychic equilibrium they establish. This disruption is critical to how something can become available to be reworked, by becoming unbound and, perhaps, bound again differently, in different or expansive ways. This emphasis on the lytic dimensions of the work is a distinctively Laplanchean style.

I don't mean to imply that every single session has such spectacularly disruptive moments or that it should; for Laplanche, too, as for me, these moments are singular, not the majority of the session, and are oftentimes the culmination of considerable and protracted prior work. I write a lot about such experiences, especially because I am interested in the experiential dimensions of what de-translation looks like in the consulting room, which is not something that Laplanche, as far as I know, wrote about. I think that because of this emphasis it often happens to me that when colleagues come to me for supervision, they expect that I can help them produce such spectacular moments for their patients. They imagine that under my supervision they will be able to generate those moments but, in truth, what galvanizes those possibilities is long-term, good analytic work and a willingness to not work in the adaptational domain but with the economies of the sexual drive. For the most part, the work is quiet, not phantasmagoric, but very, very slow. Work that tends toward unbinding is distributed in the entire fabric of a treatment; it's in how you hold the patient's material in mind, in how the analyst refuses her own defensive coagulation of the material into something fully knowable and adaptive—Laplanche describes that as the analyst guarding her enigma. Sometimes unbinding appears before you in a distinct episodic encounter (what I've called *overwhelm* [2023]) and at others it unfurls over time. Either way, much goes into what makes the moment of unbinding what it is. When you decontextualize it, e.g., when lifting it out of a treatment to discuss a vignette, it can appear as if it resulted from an interpretation or that it was produced by a particular interaction, but that is a misunderstanding and a misreading of the theory.

BBT: This is not the question I was going to ask you, but it is related to what you just said: The question of psychoanalytic writing. You're a prolific writer and there is a particular style you have of writing. Specifically, I think that's reflected in "The Draw to Overwhelm: Consent, Risk, and the Retranslation of Enigma," the paper with the hypodermic needles. Do you think that there's a particular way of writing a case? Given that Laplanche never wrote up a case, do you think that a person who thinks with Laplanche writes up cases in a particular manner, where there is a sort of openness to them? How would you think about psychoanalytic writing in this way, as compared to the way Klein, etc., wrote up a case?

AS: When you say it's open, what do you mean by open?

BBT: Sticking with "The Draw to Overwhelm: Consent, Risk, and the Retranslation of Enigma," there is a certain degree of it that feels unfinished. There's a quality to the case that feels unresolved. A feeling like I would like to know more. A kind of irritation, as it were, as though there's something not quite there. This is different from reading a Kleinian case write-up, for example, that has all these unconscious phantasies where you are left with the idea that this is what I would do, this is what it looks like.

AS: Oh, I see. Yes, for me, clinical writing needs to leave some things unanswered, to not try to totalize the case by acting as if it can explain everything, as if the analyst had thought of everything. I don't mean this as a writing technique but more in the sense that it should reflect the unfinished quality of the work, appreciating, respecting, even savoring the fact that no clinical work is complete or delivers a final answer. Clinical writing should also, in my opinion, leave you with a hunger, generating more questions, which I see as an aesthetic orientation to what is irreducibly opaque in any one clinical encounter. That's why I used the word "savoring" just now.

It's relevant to say here that while one of the critiques I often hear about Laplanche is that his theory is very cerebral, disembodied, and theoretical, I don't experience it this way at all. Indeed, Laplanche is quite careful when going back to Freud and rereading his texts—and what this means is that to read him, you need to know (or learn) Freud very well too. If you're going to read Laplanche deeply, you're going to have to go back and re-read Freud, if you want to get even that (seemingly smaller point) thing Laplanche mentions in passing in a footnote so you have your own sense of what he is talking about when he references Freud. This makes reading Laplanche a demanding and rigorous endeavor and it makes it appear—and feel, to some—as if it were only intellectually driven. I think this is where the critique that it is a theory that appeals to the intellect but does not address the body comes from and I understand why it seems like this to some people.

But when you don't just read him once but twice, thrice, multiple times over, as one must, in my opinion, if one is to really engage him, the stakes of what he says become more visible, you begin to see how very embodied, viscerally so—at times frighteningly so—he can be. He speaks to something similar, I think, when he says that theory needs to be seen as an experiment, because an experiment is something that you enter with some conviction not because you know it will work out but because you are determined to give it a go, and this amounts to taking risks. We are not accustomed to thinking about theory that entices us to take risks, that shows us why we might want or need to take them. When I teach him, I try to teach him this way, drawing attention to how the very process of learning his theory involves our bodies and our "souls". I also try to write this way, though "try" is misleading, perhaps, because I can't imagine writing differently. If my work feels "irritating" as you mentioned earlier—and I really like that you talked about the irritation in reading my work—it is because, hopefully, it does not shy away from what Scarfone (2023) refers to as the irritative spine of the enigmatic—irritating in the sense that it frustrates the desire to possess the other, to eliminate the other's otherness by understanding them fully, which is a form of exercising mastery over another.

My hope is that my writing works to activate this irritant of the enigmatic in the reader, to put in motion the drive movement of the *sexual* such that if one engages with the text, they could become fascinated, drawn in, "irritated." For me, Laplanche is the psychoanalytic theorist of disturbance and of disruption. His theory does not just "challenge" us, though it most certainly does that: Taking him seriously requires a revisitation of so much that psychoanalysis has become disconnected from that is radical and revolutionary. And it points to the rickety foundations of some of our most beloved and uncontested psychoanalytic concepts.

BBT: Are there particular concepts you have in mind?

AS: Interpretation, for one. In Laplanche's hands, interpretation becomes a rickety concept, more something that helps the analyst sidestep the disruption of the *sexual*, perhaps more of an effort, at times, to master the disquiet in oneself that is generated by the contact with the patient's otherness and with one's own. When somebody encounters something in the patient that unsteadies the analyst—take, for example, the analyst's encounter with variant forms of gender that may unsettle the analyst's own gender and sexuality—then interpretation can be a way of expelling that disquiet, packaging it in a formulation that is projected onto the patient, ridding the self of it.

In bringing in this example, I don't want to inflate what Laplanche says about gender and dysregulation; he is decidedly a man of his time. And he does raise points that could be used in transphobic ways, which is not to say that I see his writing as transphobic because he also gives us the tools with which to go much deeper than just doing an "inclusive psychoanalysis," which I think is a very low bar in thinking about difference.

In his paper "Gender, Sex, and the *Sexual*," in *Freud and the* Sexual, for example, which is the paper where he gives us his theory of gender acquisition, there are two appendices. He gets caught there in what is also the trope of his day: Stoller's conception of a "primary transsexual," which pertains to questions about who is, truly, trans and who isn't. The concession that some people are truly trans is a big statement for someone of his era and that it is a concession is the problem. For me, his engagement of Stoller runs counter to his own theory of gender acquisition—but this would take us too far afield now. The short version is that in the second of the two appendices of his paper, we see Laplanche being more tentative about the radicalness of his earlier-stated idea, where he's opened this extremely expansive, exciting, and also challenging to psychoanalysis's more orthodox investment in binary gender, landing on an argument that is alarmingly similar with the problematic rhetoric that trans children are trans by virtue of the "confused" messages emitted by parents who "wanted," e.g., a girl but gave birth to a child they read as male. At the end of the day, however, what matters most for me is that his work on gender forces us to reconsider our psychoanalytic foundations, which is his overall project; he does so by dethroning the primacy of biology in psychic life and by questioning the ontological primacy of the Oedipus complex, which he sees as a translational code as opposed to the most central ontological analytic. To not regard biology *or* the Oedipal complex as key to how we acquire our genders is to challenge received analytic ideas.

BBT: How could you see the paper being used to think about power, class, and race?

AS: I think that in order to think about race and class, we need some modifications in Laplanche's theory that go beyond this particular essay, though he most definitely hands us some of the tools to be able to do that (e.g., in the paper on gender we've been discussing). Without meaning to conflate categories of difference, which have different historical antecedents and quite distinct material implications, what Laplanche offers us is a way of thinking about how materials of culture are not just available as translational codes but partake also in processes of assignment. In a highly suggestive footnote, (ft 8) in Appendix II of the gender paper, he writes: "[I]n certain countries the registration of a birth may involve other categories than that of gender," such as "racial assignment ('white'), religious assignment (Catholic, Muslim, no religion, etc.), racial-religious assignment, etc. (Laplanche, 2011a, 2011b, p. 203)."

Even as the concepts of assignment and the relationships between the *sexual* and gender can be used as models to think about these other categories, one can't simply transpose racial assignment and religious assignment with gender assignment, as these involve not just personal history but also capital-"H" Histories. Still, there are useful resources here to draw on to think about race and religion as not just social categories (any more than gender is only a social category), but also as experiences that have psychic density and historical, intergenerational continuity for those who inhabit them. Critical here is the distinction between translation and introjection or internalization, as the former does not just take something in but reworks it (threading it not *into* the ego but threading the ego *through* these materials—the ego, that is, is constituted through these codes, these codes, re-worked, make up the ego) to create something distinctly personal. If you are going to step into these territories, I think you need a solid theoretical foundation in theories of racialization and histories of colonialism. Queer theory, trans studies, and queer of color critique can all help use Laplanchean ideas in ways that keep concepts alive without collapsing them into overly fixed formulations.

BBT: Related to what you brought up with the capital "H," Historical, and its relation to temporality, there is a relationship to the mytho-symbolic. How do you see that in the sense of developments in psychoanalytic theory? I'm thinking of research. There's research in the classical sense of scientific research where, for example, one has a control case. There's research where you can have a case that you follow for a very long time and conduct research in the sense of the singularity of the unconscious of that person or even child research. But I'm thinking you're saying that there is extra work required for gender. You cannot just use or apply that paper. You need to also know gender theory and trans studies, etc., to be able to do the extra legwork. I'm thinking about how one would conduct psychoanalytic research in a Laplanchean sense. At the same time, we're not applying here but taking into consideration that Laplanche has very specific set of boundaries as to what's psychoanalytic and what's not.

AS: Yes, and he explicitly addresses some of that himself, for example in *New Foundations for Psychoanalysis*, in the essay "For Psychoanalysis at the University," and, also, in *Freud and the* Sexual and his writings on extramural psychoanalysis, which discuss the need to be in conversation with other disciplines. But those disciplines cannot just be imported whole into psychoanalysis; any field outside psychoanalysis will be required to consider the critical role of the *sexual*. The *sexual* is not something other fields attend to, it is a uniquely analytic perspective and it has to do with the unique discovery and object of psychoanalysis, the infantile sexual. Gender theory, critical race theory, queer of color critique or trans studies, none of these engage infantile sexuality—nor should they! Laplanche gives us in the gender paper a way of thinking, but to think analytically about race, class, ethnicity, or religion, we need to do more work, and this work requires the analytic theorizer of these topics to be in proximity with other discourses. To put it differently, and this connects to our earlier conversation about a Laplanchean *style,* these interventions on Laplanche's end may more profitably be seen as gestures rather than as recipes that can be followed or applied. To use them, we have to do our own work and that involves the foreignness of interdisciplinary engagement. We need, that is, a non-dominative relationship with other discourses that does not try to subordinate them to psychoanalytic understanding but which allows psychoanalytic thinking to be wounded by other ideas, to be deconstructed such that it can be constructed anew. This is not a straightforward process as the dimension of the sexual needs to be considered here. But what it means is that on the level of theory-building, too, we need to be thinking about de-translation and re-translation.

I think that the whole originality, the liveliness of Laplanche's thinking, is in what it promises to break up, in creating the conditions for you (the clinician but, also, the theorist) to take the risk and assume the responsibility of putting something together on your own in the aftermath of de-translation. To put it differently, his theory is not synthetic but, rather, at its best has an unbinding effect: It is this dimension of this work that those who read him as an overly cerebral, disembodied thinker miss. The way he returns to Freud and de-links, for example, or pulls apart the logics of the death drive, pulls apart the logics of instinct, pulls apart the notion that gender is about identifying *with* a parent as opposed to being identified *by* a parent, all these require deconstructive work on the reader's part. And that deconstructive work is not only the rigorous work of renewed thinking: it is, as I've been arguing, subjectively experienced by the ego as a threat, is registered as a loss or a violence, certainly as a crisis.

BBT: I was wondering if we could return to the question of what constitutes a Laplanchean *style*.

AS: I can try to approach what I said earlier from another angle. One of Laplanche's distinguishing features is the way he thinks about the drive through the Fundamental Anthropological Situation, as something that is not driven by biology or inherited phylogenetically, but as arising through the infant's encounter with an adult other, an adult whose sexual unconscious is alien for the infant as much as it is alien to the adult themselves. What he offers us is a way to go back to an embodied

> psychoanalysis that can think about drivenness and about psychosexuality in a way that takes seriously the fact that, in the interaction with an adult other, the infant is exposed to more than they can process or assimilate, more than they can possibly coat with meaning.

In that sense, Laplanchean theory takes seriously the interaction with the other, but not on the level of two subjectivities encountering one another; nor does he see a one-to-one correspondence between what the other brings to us and how that affects us, as some schools of psychoanalysis focus on. He is more interested in "the reality of the message" than the message itself, which is another way of saying that he is more interested in enigma and in the dimension of psychic reality than in psychological reality (what experience the ego has, what the attachment relation is, etc.). He does not reject the importance of the latter; he is just more focused on how the energetic disruption of enigma, what he called the "noise" on the communication line, has the quality of interrupting something, upturning things.

This enables analysts who had moved away from thinking about the drive—because work around it had become too rigid, cultivating a fearful attitude to the drive as something that needed to be tamed—to find a way back to thinking about the drivenness of psychic life. He gives us a drive that is part of the animating force of psychic life, not only (or mostly) a force that threatens to upend civilization, as was one of Freud's later concerns about the drive. But this is a drive that traffics in enigma, that is actually constituted by an anarchic force that can never be known or controlled, that can never be eliminated. For me, this is key to what makes for a Laplanchean *style*: The acceptance of the fact that there are things about us, about others, that can never be conquered through knowledge, insight, or understanding.

Laplanche describes this untameability as having to do with the inevitable "failure" of translation—namely, the idea that enigma can never be fully converted into something meaning-ful, that translation always partially fails to cull the strangeness of enigma, to bind its unbound energy into a representation. This "failure" is, for him, what makes us distinctively human. And as Scarfone has noted, this ineliminable dimension of otherness in everything in us is also the guarantor of our freedom (2011); this is the element in Laplanche's thinking that I think as a distinctively Laplanchean *style*, the persistence that something always escapes the grasp of translation. In forthcoming work, I put the concept of what Laplanche sees as failure under pressure using Fred Moten's work on fugitivity (2018). I argue there that while Laplanche sees the drive as resulting from failed translational processes (i.e., the ego can never fully vanquish the foreignness of the other's enigma), such a view is partial to the ego's perspective. Said differently, it is only from the viewpoint of an ego that works to fully master alterity that the very existence of the unconscious be conceived as the result of a failed operation. If, however, we work with Moten and fugitivity, we may reconceive of the unconscious and its exigency, as a resistance to being captured by translation. From this angle, we might conceive of the

Laplanchean unconscious as a perennial escape artist, an undomesticated and ineliminable wildness that refuses domestication. This recasts translational "failure" into something else; the ego's so-called failure can be thus reconceived as a lush fallout that opens us up to our dispossession. To think of our dispossession as a site of possibility when self-possession is so often promoted as the site of agency challenges much of psychoanalytic thinking. To me, this is part of the wildly renewed thinking Laplanche's theory opens us up to.

The other thing that Laplanche gives us, which I think is also incredibly important, is that by talking about how translation constitutes the ego, and about how repression and translation are simultaneous events, we're offered a way of being able to speak of what is at the origin of our subjectivation without having to assume essences or ontologies, and sparing us from the snare of etiology or causation. The implications of this intervention are monumental. To explain: as we know, when the child translates, she treats enigma (not in the sense of curing or eliminating it but in the sense of subjecting it to a treatment) a process by which both the ego *and* the child's unconscious are constituted (the former as the result of translation, the latter as the result of primal repression). Because, as Scarfone (2023) has pointed out, the ego is subjected in the après-coup to processes of narcissistic closure, what this means is that translation is retrospectively experienced as perception or memory, that is, not as something that the subject created but as something always already there, something that the ego merely discovered! This, by the way, is what the patient and the analyst "discover" in the course of analysis—not something originary but what was at the origin of the subject's formation!

BBT: There were a couple things you brought up that make me think of content passed down through the generations. Could you discuss intergenerational transmission, and how it is conceived of in Laplanche's theory?

AS: The question of intergenerational transmission is, I think, one of the most knotted and difficult ones in the reading of Laplanche—especially so, perhaps, for relational theorists. It is not uncommon to interpret Laplanche as if he were saying that enigma is the quizzical way by which messages/meanings/dissociated material/historical legacies/nonverbally communicated experiences are transmitted across the generations from adult to child. For example, colleagues new to Laplanche will often express relief about how the notion of enigma helps them "grasp" how intergenerational transmission happens: Not through osmosis but through the enigmatic transfer, a transfer which has to do with the nonverbal dispatch of adult material onto the child.

Laplanche, however, never speaks about the transfer of content. For him, enigma is not a concealed communication, an invisible, hidden text behind a visible text, but, rather, the perturbation and the disruption in the communication line, the interference with the adaptational line.

Importantly, then, the question that comes up in thinking about intergenerational transmission: where to situate intergenerational transport in the Laplanchean model? For me intergenerational transmission and the passing down of, for example racial or religious trauma—in, say, a family that comes from a historically oppressed or traumatized group, e.g., a Black family with a history of slavery, or a Jewish family with a Holocaust history, or an Arab family with roots in occupied Palestine—may be best understood as occurring through the very codes that are made available for a child to translate. These codes appear as structures of affect—they may, indeed, be nonverbal (e.g., they are not always or necessarily openly discussed); but more so than that, they are elaborate systems of representation. Consider, for instance, phrases like "Never again," or, the Palestinian notion of "sumud" or the idea of "Black excellence." All of these phrases by far exceed the meaning of the words themselves; they carry in them an aura of something else, a sense that they call up more than what their words mean when strung together. Said differently, such phrases have baked within them entire lives of history and of the past, chronicles of survival which are shared by the group but which are also very particular to the adults who are rearing the child—and can become translational vessels through which the child's ego then becomes constituted (see also, Saketopoulou and Pellegrini, 2023, pp. 62–74). This is how history becomes embodied, experienced as having been always in one's body even if one has not personally experienced.

For me, it makes sense to think about intergenerational transmission as involving a set of codes that is specific to a culture, to a historical moment, to a chronological lineage in a family. In a recent conversation, Dominique Scarfone and I thought about intergenerational transmission through the use of Walter Benjamin's notion of the aura (in Scarfone, 2023, pp. 113–116, 234–235). Some words, he wrote, "might have been 'loaded' with an energy" that the child senses but cannot understand, words that operate as "a live wire in the family narrative, even if, as we may suppose, the word could be spoken without constant awareness of the tragic story it referred to" (Scarfone, 2023, p. 114). This is an excellent exposition of how trauma ripples through the generations not by unconscious transmission but through the very materials that the child will rely on to constitute her translations and, therefore, her sense of herself and of her history.

BBT: Since we're on the topic of intergenerational transmission of trauma, are there other notions of Laplanche's theory that you find are misread here in the United States? Or that the relational tradition misreads?

AS: I think his notion of a *sexual* death drive that preserves the inseparability of binding and unbinding is one of those elements. Since Freud separated out these two drives (and Laplanche, as you know, gives us a very detailed and interesting account of how that happened in his 1997 paper *The So-Called Death Drive: A Sexual Drive*), it's been nearly impossible to put the two back together. It's hard to return, that is, to a *sexual* that is also anarchic without imputing motivational dimensions to this anarchy (e.g., of destructiveness or of repetition compulsion).

On another point, and I am not sure if this is exactly a misreading of Laplanche per se, I would say that the question of how to apply Laplanchean theory or how to think clinically with Laplanche in the consulting room misunderstands what a Laplanchean *style* is about. For me, it betrays a certain kind of anxiety that, in fact, the theory itself generates because of, as we discussed earlier, how committed it is to the irreducible opacity inherent in the human condition. Oftentimes, the wish to articulate a Laplanchean method or to locate this or that concept in the clinical material is driven by an anxiety to master the theory, to command it. It's not that I believe that Laplanchean concepts cannot be identified in the clinical moment; it's more about how that exercise is sometimes deployed as a response to the difficulty of the theory. This difficulty is not only conceptual (we talked already about how well one needs to know Freud to work with Laplanche), it also requires deep and genuine respect for the unknowability of the unconscious, an ongoing resistance to the inclination to interpret the unconscious in the way one translates a text from one language to the other.

BBT: I know you wanted to talk about *après-coup*.

AS: Yes, thank you. I wanted to speak about that in the context of de-translation and re-translation. We talked already about how translation does not offer some veridical rendering of adult communication but, rather, "treats" the other's enigmatic incursion by coating it with meaning (sourced from the mytho-symbolic realm as mediated by the adult). Under certain circumstances (e.g., in an analytic treatment), these bindings can come undone, can become de-translated, which is the de-linking of the unbound energy of enigma from its representational coating. In such cases, the ego will quickly rush in to treat the newly free enigma, generating new translations; these re-translations are not guaranteed to be better, though one hopes they show some progress.

I would argue, however, that a temporal quality is also at work with processes of de- and re-translation.

To explain what I mean, let me bring an example. Let us imagine, a subject who is atypically gendered. And let us also imagine that in the aftermath of the proliferation of transgender discourses they come to wonder if they may themselves be trans (as opposed to, say, being a feminine gay man). This new possibility could retroactively make the original translation of their gender through a binary form into an intromissive injunction: In the *après-coup*, that is, what in real time had amounted to a reliance on the then-available translational tools of binary gender could, after the fact of these social shifts, retroactively reinscribe the original binary choice into an injunction to translate in a binary way, making it traumatic, that is, in the *après-coup*. To say this differently, some trans subjects may only retroactively come to experience the initial mandate that they arrange themselves into a neat male/

> female classificatory divide as traumatic. This is different than saying that the experience was traumatic all along and only became possible to register as such when a trans person came to realize that transgender life and embodiment may be viable possibilities. What distinguishes that from the workings of the *après-coup* is that the injunction to normative gender may become traumatic *after* discursive shifts of gender as multiple have occurred and *because of them;* these shifts, that is, may act as the second coup in the après-coup. Said differently, one's own gender translation can become traumatic only after—and because of—the encounter with enlarged possibilities afforded by new translational codes around gender. Why? Because that revisitation can in the present time generate excitations that reopen enigma, but which, through today's translational gender possibilities, render the binary gender options of the past into interdictions to translate as anything but binary and fixed, restrictive. My larger point is not gender-specific; I am only using gender to elaborate the following idea: that, for some subjects, cultural shifts can, in the *après-coup,* spin implantation into the orbit of intromission.

The scrambled temporality of the *après-coup* means that it is not until *after* cultural shifts permit the emergence of novel translational possibilities that the restrictiveness of earlier translational codes (what, via Aulagnier, we discussed earlier as the violence of the translational codes themselves) may come to be experienced as violent in the first place—therefore becoming traumatic *after* the fact. Cultural changes, in that sense, create translational funnels with wider translational possibilities (e.g., multiple genders rather than two, etc.) that could not have been furnished or imagined by the adult—because of the adult's cultural and historical situatedness, own anxieties about their own gender and sexuality, and so on. These new funnels can then, in turn, be taken up by the subject to translate anew, resulting in entirely different psychic positions which may render the original ones traumatic. This makes translation, implantation, and intromission historically contingent events, tying them together with questions of temporality, of the passage of time and of chance rather than being, as they are often presented to be, ontologically different processes.

BBT: If we can speak about exigency, and what Laplanche leaves open….

AS: What is exigent for Laplanche is the unconscious. For him it is this that is *the* object of psychoanalysis, it is this that always eludes us. For Laplanche, the unconscious is not meaning-ful but, as we said earlier, the result of translational failure or, in my mind, it pertains to resistance to capture. The unconscious imposes itself, it intervenes, it interrupts, it blisters through other psychic surfaces—the ego most of all. And it is impervious to other kinds of realities. It is impervious to external influence. It is impervious to psychological reality. It is impervious to

> educative or therapeutic goals. It is all these precisely because it is constituted through repression, by remaining fugitive to the psyche's efforts to "treat" enigma through the mytho-symbolic codes made available by the adult. It is because of this unremitting force that de-translations and re-translations are possible in the first place; it is the unconscious that ensures that we can be in a state of continuous becoming.

Again, as I mentioned earlier, Laplanche describes the psyche's inability to fully cull the foreignness of the unconscious as a failure. My point in bringing in Moten is to underline that the ego would always prefer to flatten enigma's perturbation; it will always want to annex the enigmatic into its territories. Enigma's energetically insubordinate fugitivity guarantees, however, that unbound energy will always manage to escape the ego's despotic command over what is centrifugal in psychic life. It is in this constant spirit of escape, in its persistence and imperviousness to being fully domesticated, that we might situate the exigency of the unconscious. Exigency captures this unsuppressible quality. Think, for example, how ego psychology sets as its goal to bring the unconscious under the rubric of the ego ("Where id was there shall ego be"), to substitute the anarchic elements of unconscious life with measured and mature ego functions. In these models, the unconscious is seen as a danger, as posing a risk to the ego's stability (aka, threatening its full dominion over the apparatus of the soul), whereas for Laplanche, the exigency of the unconscious is what psychoanalysis distinctively concerns itself with.

BBT: What are some aspects of Laplanche's theory that you feel he doesn't complete? Also, if we could return to the question about what research in the Laplanchean sense could look like.

AS: I am not sure if we're using the word "research" in the same way, but what I am thinking is that research would involve taking seriously the irritative spine in his own ideas, and pursuing those—seeing what else can open up, even be blown open, if we do not avoid engaging them. I use this language purposefully, of blowing things open, because even as Laplanche understood himself as merely buttressing the Freudian foundation, I think he has done much more than that. Continuing to work with his ideas, even stretching them, can blast open some doors—and the violence in the words I am using is deliberate, chosen to capture the level of disarray and dysregulation this can cause. This is not about being destructive, it's about—I am now forgetting the word in English, it's about what remains when there is an earthquake and everything collapses but the door remains, what's that word…?

BBT: The frame.

AS: Yes, the frame! There are some basic structures in his thinking that are the robust, weight bearing columns, that remain—for example, his important distinction between the drive and instinct.

This is well known now, but to explain what I mean: In translating Freud, James Strachey makes some decisions about which Laplanche remains skeptical—when it comes to the terms "drive" and "instinct." For Laplanche, this is quite consequential because "instinct" should be reserved specifically for processes that have to do with the biological character of human capacities, whereas the "drive" is specifically psychic; it becomes constituted through the failure of translation which, nevertheless, keeps pressing, an ongoing pressure that is exerted on the psyche to translate material that has remained enigmatic.

Laplanche fleshes out this distinction in an important paper where he discusses the differences between these two terms (2011a). He points out there their features and makes a compelling argument for why we should consistently adopt this distinctive terminology for these two different processes: "instincts" work towards specific aims. For example, the sexual instinct moves toward orgasm, it moves toward release, toward climax. Whereas the *sexual* drive does not. "Drives" are not teleologically driven in the same way; they are driven by the principle of escalation. These two operate, thus, on very distinctive economic regimes.

In this case, the drive and the instinct are part of the frame I was referring to earlier—they stay standing no matter what gets blown open. What can you do with these standing principles? Research, for me, is to follow the exigency of the questions that one cannot not ask! For example, if the drive is not teleologically driven, how do we think about contingency and chance? Contingency and chance are not questions that have interested psychoanalysis very much; the focus has been more on determinism—actually, *over*determinism. But Laplanche's distinction between drive and instinct helps us to ask questions of that sort; If the instinct has a preordained, built-in endpoint (orgasm, satisfaction, etc.), what about the drive's escalation—what does it escalate to and what stops it from continuing to do so forever?

My point is not only that those questions become possible because of Laplanche's insistence on differentiating the two. It is also to say that whatever research you do in this domain is framed by this distinction. To say this a bit more concretely (though perhaps, also, a bit more clumsily), there is no room per se behind that frame; the whole idea is that one might construct a new room each time one seriously, and with theoretical rigor, engages the frame to explore further. The incitement to think is there precisely because Laplanche has left some things unfinished, which is another way of saying that there's something enigmatic in the theory itself that can propel us as thinkers to engage with it, to create more theory, to do our own research. To engage with him as somebody who is putting forth a set of aporias—that, while thoughtful and well-framed, remain still aporetic, enigmatic as opposed to puzzles that can be solved—is to be propelled to continue the process of theorization.

The last thing that I would mention regarding research relates to a Laplanchean idea that to many analysts might sound counterintuitive. Where most of our colleagues understand our work as about being attentive to our patients' wounds by means of witnessing and holding and helping repair, Laplanche sees the analyst's work quite differently: As being about keeping the wound open. This is something he mentions in a couple of places in his work, albeit mostly as a passing thought. I say "passing thought" not to imply that it's unimportant to him, but precisely to invoke this image of a frame without a whole structure attached to it, as he never fully develops that idea into something more elaborated. In my own research, I've taken this idea of traumatophiia very seriously and have expounded it to a full-fledged concept. To me, the re-direction of psychoanalysis towards keeping the wound open extremely intriguing: He means, of course, to create the circumstances for enigma to be reopened in the encounter with an analyst who is guarding her own enigma and who is minding the asymmetry of the relationship. The wound, we might say, is what lies beneath the scabbing over that translation provides. This is an ontological wound that is related to our very being, as opposed to a wound in the sense of having been hurt or injured. It is in this context, and only in very few places, that he names the concept of "traumatophilia," and to me this is one of the most exciting domains in Laplanchean thought, which is why I have dedicated so much space to it in my own writings.

I'm personally as grateful for what Laplanche has given us as I am thankful for the things that he has necessarily left unfinished: He has given us new foundations for psychoanalysis, and this, to me, feels like an invitation, an opening that also carries a responsibility. A responsibility toward a psychoanalysis that is devoted to exploring psychic reality without getting lost in psychological reality, a psychoanalysis that follows the exigency of the sexual unconscious, that remains at a mindful distance from enigma without trying to colonize or apprehend it, a psychoanalysis which respects the fact that contingency and chance are operative in the mechanism of the *après-coup*. For me, Laplanche has given us a path that is as trailblazing as it is replete with an infinite number of unexplored paths. He leaves it to us to dare venturing into them!

Notes

1 "In the Laplanchean framework, 'translation,' despite the word's misleading implication, does not refer to some veridical rendering of what the adult non-verbally communicated to the child but to the way in which the child 'treats' the enigma of the adult's sexual unconscious by 'coating' it—as Scarfone puts it— with meaning."

2 While Laplanche speaks mostly about the mytho-symbolic world, Aulagnier is also in ongoing conversation with the political theorist Cornelius Castoriadis. This opens space for us to be thinking about how the mytho-symbolic world is a political one.

Bibliography

Aulagnier, P. (1984). *The violence of interpretation*. Routledge, New Library of Psychoanalysis.

Laplanche, J. (2011a). *Freud and the sexual*. NY: The Unconscious in Translation.

Laplanche, J. (2011b). Gender, sex, and the sexual. In Jonathan House (ed.), *Freud and the sexual: Essays, 2000–2006* (pp. 167–209). The Unconscious in Translation.

Laplanche, J., & House, J. (2016). *New foundations for psychoanalysis*. NY: The Unconscious in Translation.

Laplanche, J., & Mehlman, J. (2015). *Between seduction and inspiration: Man*. NY: The Unconscious in Translation.

Moten, F. (2018). *Consent not to be a single being: Stolen life*. Durham: Duke University Press.

Saketopoulou, A. (2019). The draw to overwhelm: Consent, risk, and the retranslation of enigma. *Journal of the American Psychoanalytic Association, 67*(1), 133–167.

Saketopoulou, A. (2023). *Sexuality beyond consent: Risk, race, traumatophilia*. New York: NYU Press.

Saketopoulou, A. & Pellegrini, A. (2023). *Gender without Identity*. New York: Unconscious in Translation Press.

Saketopoulou, A. (forthcoming). Exigent sadism: Austerity logics and the anti-reparative turn. *Social Text,* 116. https://doi.org/10.1177/0003065119830088

Scarfone, D. (2011). Repetition: Between presence and meaning. *Canadian Journal of Psychoanalysis / Revue Canadienne de Psychanalyse, 19*(1), 70–86.

Scarfone, D. (2023). *The reality of the message: Psychoanalysis in the wake of Jean Laplanche*. The Unconscious in Translation.

Afterword—Hélène Tessier

Saint Paul University (Ottawa), Canadian Psychoanalytic Society and Institute (Montréal French Branch), Montréal, Canada

This book is the result of the author/editor Bryan Batista-Thomas's deep interest in Laplanche's work and thought. For many years, he has taken part in study groups with experts in Laplanche's work and studied it in depth. He worked with me on issues pertaining to metapsychology and the clinical implications of Laplanche's thought. In this context, he became interested in the uses of Laplanche's thought in the work of psychoanalysis, those who were involved in his work, and how they were relying on it in different ways. Following his own interests, Bryan envisioned this book as a way to make Laplanche's work, and the way it developed in different countries and cultural environments, better known to English-speaking readers.

Laplanche underlined how problematic fragmentation and lack of communication among scientists could apply to any discipline, and psychoanalysts were no exception. He regretted that, often, scientific meetings in psychoanalysis could only propose juxtapositions of contributions. He wrote:

> ...[W]e shall go much further if psychoanalysis is not to become a corpse. There is an urgent need for debate among those who want to debate. It is time for texts and thesis to reply to each other with a rigor that does not exclude tolerance, rigor with respect to ideas, tolerance with respect to others....
>
> (Countercurrent, in *Freud and the* Sexual*, Essays 2000–2006*, p. 97)

This book invites us to reflect on Laplanche's thought by "amplifying differences" in the interpretation of his work. It is indeed a worthwhile endeavor, since it emphasizes how Laplanche's thought becomes a fruitful soil for creative thinking. New developments arising from Laplanche's work do not necessarily follow the path of Laplanche's own theory. Laplanche's thought arose from debates with Freud as well as with post-Freudians. It still stimulates debates and does not respond well to being silenced by arguments of authority, whether coming from Freud, Lacan, other prominent post-Freudians, or even another Laplanchean concept taken out of the context of the general history of his work and ideas.

Therefore, as much as it is important to acknowledge the differences between new uses and understanding of Laplanche's theory, it is also necessary to debate with them. The issue is not to force new ideas to be in line with Laplanche's thought. It is simply to ask ourselves whether such interpretations or elaborations respect the founding principles of Laplanche's theory and, whatever the outcome of this analysis, whether those founding principles are determinant in our conception of psychoanalysis.

In earlier papers, I had the opportunity to present what were the main principles of Laplanche's work, which makes it invaluable for the future of psychoanalysis, if psychoanalysis as a specific field and a specific method, as well as metapsychology as a scientific theory, is to survive at all. I will mention some of them here, hoping that they can serve as relevant tools to evaluate what is worth preserving in Laplanche's work.

Laplanche's work is based on a specific anthropology, in other words, on a conception of the human being and of the conditions necessary for becoming human. One of these conditions is sexualization, through the formation of the repressed sexual unconscious. Laplanche's anthropology is guided by the idea of a human capable of transformation, living in a world which is also transformable, because both the world and the human being are considered in a human, historical perspective. This transformation is possible because sexualization, for Laplanche, results from a historical event, primary repression, implying humans and human processes. What is done by humans can be changed by human means.

This anthropology directs the epistemological choices in which Laplanche's work is grounded. One of these choices is a very strict delimitation of the epistemological field of psychoanalysis. The border of psychoanalysis, according to him, has to be drawn by the line that separates infantile sexuality from self-preservation. Fantasy, in its relationship with excitation, is, according to him, a concrete way to define the object of psychoanalysis.

Laplanche was totally committed to the "Copernican revolution" in psychoanalysis. By this expression, he refers to the primacy of the other in the formation of infantile sexuality. Infantile sexuality is not inborn. It does not come from self-preservation or bodily functions. It has to come from a material that is already sexual, and this material is the unconscious sexual fantasy of the concrete, historical adult who takes care of the child. This external otherness, through primary repression, becomes an internal otherness that constitutes the repressed sexual unconscious.

The primacy of the other, in Laplanche's metapsychology, revolves around two concepts that both involve the other: seduction and translation. They both imply not only another human but also messages, an essential category of Laplanche's metapsychology. Messages in Laplanche's epistemology are not reducible to their meaning or as carriers of information, as they are in communication theories. In addition, they cannot be confused with the "speech acts" of performative theories. Messages signify something, but they signify it to someone. They are addressed. They interpellate; they "make a sign" ("*font signe*"). They always represent another for someone.

Laplanche's epistemology is resolutely humanist. He has argued against postmodern and deconstructionist theories. His description of psychoanalysis as an "anti-hermeneutics" and his definition of *après-coup* as a specific form of human, interpersonal temporality are both a rebuttal of Heideggerian positions.

Laplanche finds his place in the line of humanist semiotics. Like Saussure, Laplanche postulates that, in science,[1] the global precedes the local, a proposition which has been rejected in the now dominant postmodern uses of interpretations. In this respect, it does not render justice to Laplanche's own way of theorizing—to interpret his work by isolating a sentence, a concept, or even a paper, out of context or out of his thought as it globally developed over the years. He saw metapsychology as a scientific endeavor which involved the aim to formulate some truth about its object.

Laplanche's anthropology describes the human being as an interpreter. Meaning is central in Laplanche's thought. He sees the sexual unconscious as the circulation of "non-meaning," whereas he defines the ego as an auto-theorization and an auto-historization. Forces at play in psychical conflict have to be understood in this perspective. Though painful, conflict is the motor of transformation. The psychoanalytic process, in the best conditions, fosters the analysand's quest for freer, less rigid, more encompassing translations and auto-historizations.

I argue that Laplanche's thought can serve as safeguards against, or at least as a tool to counter, the attacks on meaning and symbolization that are at work in the current cultural conditions. To be able to serve as such, a re-centering on Laplanche's basic principles is, in my view, necessary.

Note

1 Of course, not in the psychoanalytic method.

Bibliography

Laplanche, J. (2011). *Freud and the sexual*. The Unconscious in Translation.

Index

Note: Page numbers followed by "n" refer to end notes